Praise for
Character and Caring: A Pandemic
Year in Medical Education

Character and Caring: A Pandemic Year in Medical Education is a powerful and timely collection that provides important insights into what all of us in academic medicine were experiencing. The essays capture the challenges, the joys, the grief, and the determination that impacted our communities. Some of the words you read will break your heart, others will inspire and give you hope. They are all compelling.

I invite faculty and staff, students, residents and fellows everywhere to read, reflect and learn from these extraordinary snapshots.

-Aviad Haramati, PhD
Professor, Integrative Physiology and Medicine and Director of the Center for Innovation and Leadership in Education (CENTILE) at Georgetown University Medical Center

This moving, informative, and inspiring collection of personal stories, observations, and commentaries, captures the angst and desperation, as well as the resiliency and creativity of individuals and institutions to meet challenges never anticipated. This compilation serves as a vital record of a unique period in the history of our nation and academic medicine, when there was an urgent need to confront and change the present, while keeping a hopeful eye on the future. Through the eyes of learners, clinicians, educators, and researchers, one gains a perspective not often shared and experiences how these resourceful individuals adapted to new realities even while dealing with their own personal issues. The reader gets close enough to experience the fear, confusion, restlessness, sadness, grief, anger, pride, joy, hope, courage, and love that have been hallmarks of the response to the pandemic and national issues over the past year.

As I read this book, I felt myself reliving many of the events with a clarity and understanding one gets from "having been there." The writers are part of my extended academic family who radically and creatively changed their practices, educational routines, research, and outreach in an exceedingly short period of time. As individuals, mothers, fathers, sisters, brothers, children, partners, and friends, together we have felt the loss of loved ones as well as frustration of dealing with realities that could have been different.

Through thoughtful narratives, this book captures the realities of a tumultuous year and provides an inspiring insight into how academic medicine can rise to better understand, confront, and meet today's challenges while preparing and adapting to those of tomorrow.

-John E. Prescott, MD
Former Chief Academic Officer at the Association of American Medical Colleges (AAMC), founding Chair of the Department of Emergency Medicine and former Dean at the West Virginia University School of Medicine

"No words can describe this experience," writes one contributor to this stunning volume. The words mount—isolation, grief, danger, rage, intimacy, disbelief, loss, activism, gravity, loneliness, despair, power, promise. As we readers read, we undergo our own COVID-19 experiences, refracted through the *Transformational Times* archives. MCW and Kern Institute's visionaries captured this multitude of voices in the immediacy of their utterance and now harvest the words in a lasting act of healing. Words *are* enough—they are all we have.

-Rita Charon, MD, PhD
Bernard Schoenberg Professor of Social Medicine and Professor of Medicine, Chair of the Department of Medical Humanities and Ethics, and Executive Director of the Columbia Narrative Medicine Program at the Columbia Vagelos College of Physicians & Surgeons

This collection of sixty-two essays, stories, and creative responses caused me to pause, reflect, think, feel, and discuss difficult matters with colleagues and family. As we toil each day in academic medicine with the tyranny of the urgent--especially the coronavirus pandemic and racism in our communities--it is easy for us to get caught up in the clinical, scientific, organizational, and political aspects of the matters at hand. Inside, though, I believe each of us is also experiencing deep and profound feelings. These emotions are very personal, and I am pleased that so many members of the Medical College of Wisconsin (MCW) community shared their stories. These narratives, which reflect the feelings and emotions of the time, have been gathered and recorded skillfully and thoughtfully.

The diversity of contributors greatly enriches these perspectives, as does the dozen or so reflections from Kern Institute Director Adina Kalet, MD, MPH, which discuss how contemporary issues intersect with medical education in admissions, residency interviews, childcare, and work-life balance. Her thoughtful and informed contributions add a punctuating consistency to the broad and diverse perspectives offered in the collected works.

As I entered each section of the book, I found myself enthusiastically anticipating what the season's authors would offer in the pages ahead. I was not disappointed by their impressive contributions.

As future generations are taught about this current period in our history, *Character and Caring: A Pandemic Year in Medical Education* will become a reference that explores the very important human perspectives that were shaped by the science and politics of our current time.

-Michael L. Good, MD
Dean, Spencer Fox Eccles School of Medicine and Senior Vice President for Health Sciences at the University of Utah

Character and Caring: A Pandemic Year in Medical Education

Essays, Stories, and Creative Responses to a Unique Time in History Selected from the Kern Institute's *Transformational Times* Newsletter

Editors: Adina Kalet, Bruce H. Campbell, Wendy Peltier, Kathlyn Fletcher, Julia Schmitt, Erin Weileder, Rachel Keane

Ten|16
PRESS

www.ten16press.com - Waukesha, WI

For information, please contact:

Ten|16
P R E S S

www.ten16press.com
Waukesha, WI

Cover design by Kaeley Dunteman
Cover Image Credit: Omer Yildiz | unsplash.com
Interior Imagery Credit: Craig Whitehead, Clay Banks, Steven
Cornfield, Jose Castillo, Parker Johnson | unsplash.com

The editors have made every effort to ensure that the information
within this book was accurate at the time of publication. The
editors do not assume and hereby disclaim any liability to any
party for any loss, damage, or disruption caused by errors
or omissions, whether such errors or omissions result from
accident, negligence, or any other cause.

Patients' names and identifying information have been changed
throughout to maintain HIPAA compliance. To find the
original essays, many of which contain references and/or links
to additional reading, go to https://bit.ly/3lN2iU8.

**The views and content expressed are those of the individual
authors and not those of the Medical College of Wisconsin or
the Kern Family Foundation.**

TABLE OF CONTENTS

Foreword from
Christopher Stawski, PhD

The Kern Family Foundation's mission is to empower the rising generation of Americans to build flourishing lives anchored in strong character, inspired by quality education, driven by an entrepreneurial mindset, and guided by the desire to create value for others. Centered in this mission and recognizing the need to train for medical professionals of character, the Foundation worked with the leaders of the Medical College of Wisconsin to establish the Robert D. and Patricia E. Kern Institute for the Transformation of Medical Education in 2017. Since that time, the Kern Institute has grown to become a center of gravity within the MCW community and beyond in efforts to advance character, caring, and competence in the training of physicians through its multiple programs and events supporting faculty, residents, staff, and students.

When the effects of the pandemic began to reach all of us by March 2020, it became clear that healthcare professionals would be at the forefront of efforts not only to use their skills to care for patients who had become ill with COVID-19, but they would also be carriers of the existential challenges of practicing their craft amidst uncertainty regarding treatment, the dangers to their own lives and others that this would pose, and bearing witness to the pain of patients and families suffering with the effects of the disease. In answering the call to be present during this time of emergency and tragedy, the Kern Institute asked how it could provide a way to connect and support the medical education community— to provide a human touch—when in-person contact was understood to be threatening to one's life.

The *Transformational Times*, though initially developed as a response to this concern to stay connected and create a shared space during the initial stages of the pandemic, has become an outlet for communicating character, caring, and competence in medical education through engaging storytelling and meaningful reflection that speaks to the lived experience of those working in the healthcare ecosystem. Since its creation, it has found its voice by highlighting the thoughts and perspectives of those in the MCW community during this challenging moment. From the weekly "Director's Corner" essays from Adina Kalet and guest contributors, to the thoughtful essays that are penned by different authors for each issue, to the Poetry Corner that opens our eyes to different ways of seeing, the *Transformational Times* seeks both to raise issues of importance for our attention in medical education, while also prompting reflection and sparking joy in its readers.

Character and Caring: A Pandemic Year in Medical Education shares a sampling of some of the essays and contributions from the *Transformational Times* since its beginnings in Spring 2020. It traces the seasons of a community reflecting in the moment on questions, concerns, and struggles among those who are striving to do their best to live up to the highest ideals of the medical profession. I have often been moved by the stories and perspectives that have been shared and have learned more about how to be both a person and a professional who exhibits character and caring along the way. I have also had the good fortune of contributing to the *Transformational Times* and have been grateful and honored to participate in the process. Much credit goes to the Kern Institute community for embracing this outlet as a forum to communicate with others their experiences, vulnerabilities, and expertise, in hopes that it will have an impact on each reader. Along the way, it provides an opportunity for all who engage to reflect on their purpose and calling as a medical professional, and in doing so become part of a wider community with shared commitments.

I hope you enjoy the selections contained in this volume and I look forward to the continuing work of the Kern Institute in its efforts to advance character, caring, and competence in medical education.

Christopher Stawski, PhD
Senior Program Director and Senior Fellow,
Kern Family Foundation

Foreword from
Joseph E. Kerschner, MD, FACS, FAAP

At the Medical College of Wisconsin (MCW), educating healers has always been at the center of our values and raison d'être. While many hospitals and institutions provide outstanding healthcare, precious few take up the challenge and the calling to teach tomorrow's physicians! MCW has always felt enormously privileged to be, among other things, a medical school that tackles the important work of educating the next generation of physicians.

Over the decades, MCW has dedicated itself to becoming a leader in the world of medical education. Coinciding with our growing expertise was a generous gift from the Kern Family and Kern Family Foundation that established the Robert D. and Patricia E. Kern Institute for the Transformation of Medical Education in 2017. This gift—the largest personal gift in MCW's history and one of the largest gifts ever supporting medical education—quickly catalyzed groups of educators and researchers across the country to focus on reimaging medical education, guided by the Kern Institute's imperatives of educating a healthcare workforce exemplified by Character, Caring, and Competence. It is a daunting and exhilarating prospect.

Just as the process was gaining momentum, the pandemic shut down institutions across America. Any gains our educational transformation work had made might have been lost as systems retreated to old paradigms. There were threats to education, equity, and population health. The future was (and remains) uncertain.

Those were dark days. On March 20, 2020, thanks to the vision of the Kern Institute's Director, Adina Kalet, MD, MPH, the *Transformational Times* newsletter was launched, hoping to shine a light into the void.

I have enjoyed reading the newsletter, and each week's contributions have engaged and challenged me. As the months passed, I became convinced that colleagues outside of our MCW family would benefit from reading the thoughts, insights, and visions reflected in the best of the essays. Thus, we offer the collected highlights in *Character and Caring: A Pandemic Year in Medical Education.*

I hope that this volume sparks conversations and transformation as we work to educate and inspire the next generation of medical students. Education is what we do. Creating the best system possible is our goal and will be our legacy.

If you are reading this, you are already committed to the task. I wish you all the success in your journeys ahead!

Joseph E. Kerschner, MD
    Provost and Executive Vice President
    The Julia A. Uihlein, MA, Dean of the Medical
    College of Wisconsin School of Medicine

Introduction

The *Transformational Times*:
A Newsletter Born of the Pandemic

Before March 2020, the Robert D. and Patricia E. Kern Institute for the Transformation of Medical Education was intent on organizing faculty, staff, and students from medical schools across the country to envision the future of medical education. The institute's director, Adina Kalet, MD, MPH, was shaping conversations around how curricula must evolve to create a character-driven and caring medical workforce. Leaders collaborated through face-to-face meetings, at conferences, and in the hallways. Relationships were created and plans laid. The task was daunting, but given the lofty goals and the obvious need, the participants were engaged.

Then, in March 2020, everything changed.

Reports of the novel coronavirus, SARS-CoV-2, and the disease now known as COVID-19 began to dominate the news. The arrival of the virus, which had rapidly made its way from China to Europe and then the US, was met with alarm. By March 10, 2020, restaurants, travel, entertainment venues, places of worship, and businesses began shuttering. Schools, including our own Medical College of Wisconsin, closed their campuses and sent students home. Giant educational machines sputtered, heaved, and ground to a halt. The silence was deafening.

It was an eerily quiet moment in history. We wondered, What response should we have? What risks will our friends who are sent to the front-line face? Are we overreacting? Or not being cautious enough? Will we be able to "do this" for more than a few weeks?

Within days, new voices emerged, creating a cacophony of opinion and conflicting views. Medical students sat at home as faculty rushed to figure out how to create meaningful virtual sessions. Distance learning classes went from concept to reality within a few days to offer students opportunities to learn and interact. Medical schools in hard-hit cities like New York graduated their students early so they could care for the sick and dying. Physicians, nurses, and staff, especially in the emergency rooms and intensive care units, worried about their own health, the risks to their families, the rising death toll, and their inability to offer a moment of healing touch to the dying. Nurses and doctors filled social media with photos of the scars and creases on their faces and their need for more protective equipment. The country praised its brave frontline caregivers.

Within the medical community, there was anxiety unlike anything seen since the emergence of HIV/AIDS in the 1990s. Here was another disease which spread invisibly, disproportionately affected vulnerable populations, could kill healthcare workers, and for which there was no known cure.

Into this moment, the Kern Institute sought to engage the Medical College of Wisconsin. The *Transformational Times* newsletter was created to offer words of support and comfort to its readers, knowing that we were all facing an uncertain future.

The first issue of the *Transformational Times* was published after only three days of planning on March 20, 2020. The newsletter sought to be honest and timely, amplifying the voices of those who are not often heard, and sharing insights from leaders and champions. Over time, we wondered what opportunities these difficult times might offer.

Of course, in March 2020, we could never have predicted the other challenges our community and the world would soon face. We did not know about the impending importance of the Black Lives Matter movement or the worldwide social justice protests. These events became important touchstones in our lives together.

This book is broken into the five seasons—from Spring 2020 to Spring 2021—that reflect the progression of our shared experiences. As a community, we moved from fear of the unknown to fear of the known. And we grew weary.

As Dr. Kalet noted in the first newsletter,

While we have little control over this rapidly evolving situation, we can respond in community. Sometimes, the moments are dramatic, but more often they manifest as simple opportunities to express and appreciate courage, compassion, and accountability in small ways.

In this spirit, we will deliver this weekly communication highlighting caring and character amid your full inbox of technical emails. Our aim is to support and celebrate caregivers, provide a forum, and examine the role of trainees as we explore uncharted territory together.

I hope you'll find comfort and support in this weekly exchange of stories, as we celebrate caring and character during this pandemic. Please consider sharing your thoughts by responding to next week's prompt below. Thank you, stay well, and keep in touch.

We *did*—and we continue to—keep in touch. Join us as we revisit some of the most compelling essays, poems, and community responses gathered during an important and formative time in the history of our society, in medical education writ large and, in particular, at the Medical College of Wisconsin.

Adina Kalet, MD, MPH
    Director, The Robert D. and Patricia E. Kern Institute for the Transformation of Medical Education
Bruce H. Campbell, MD, FACS
Wendy Peltier, MD
Kathlyn Fletcher, MD, MA
Julia Schmitt
Erin Weileder
Rachel Keane

December, 2021

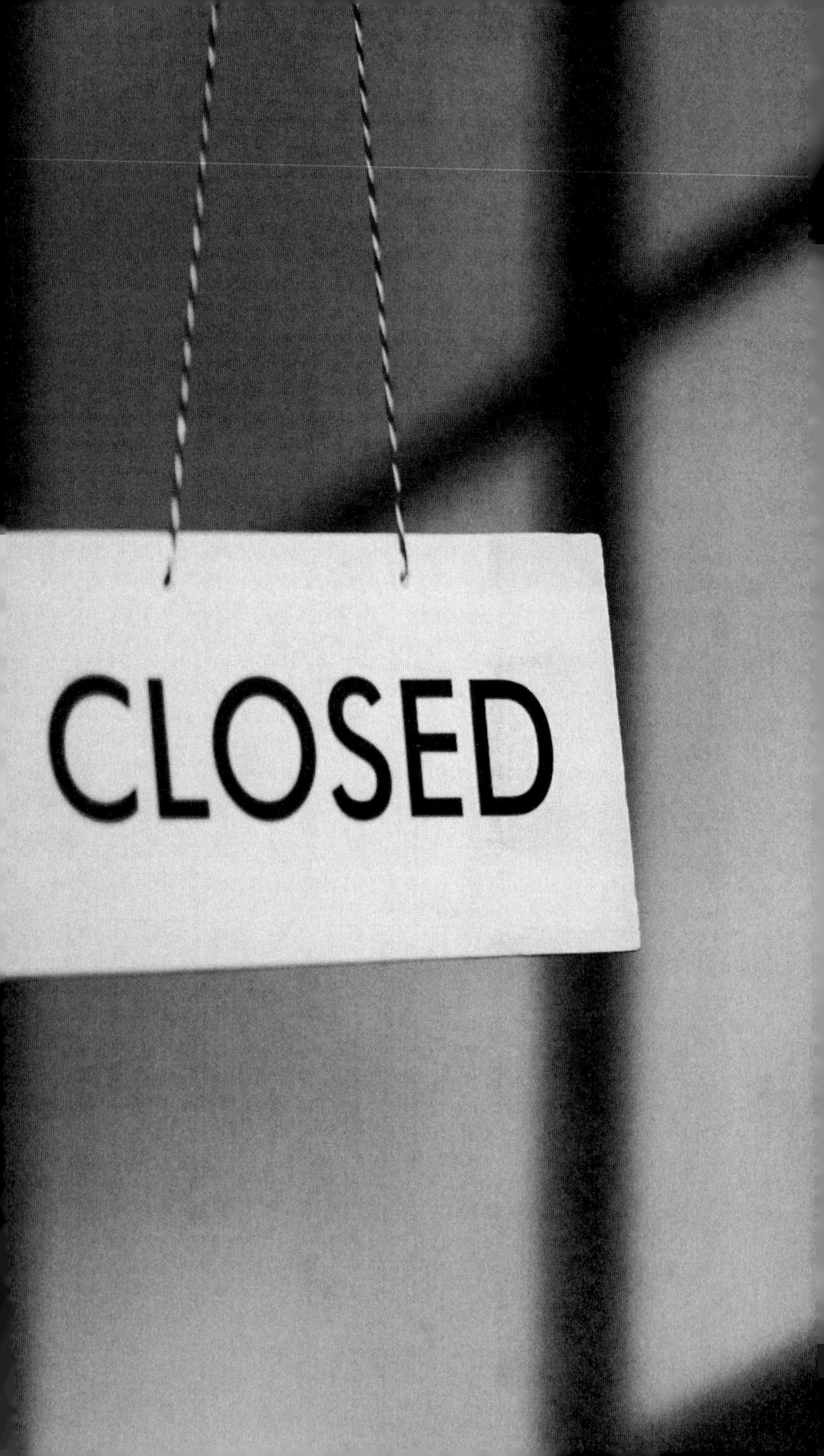
CLOSED

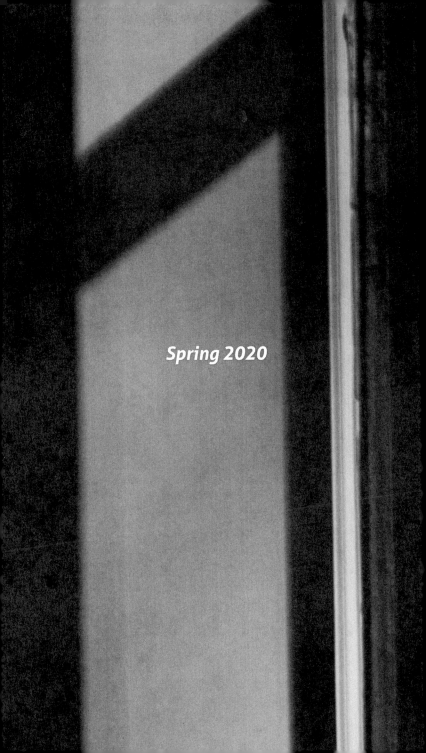

Spring 2020

Now We Wait: What it was Like to Wake up in New York City on 9/11

Adina Kalet, MD MPH

Dr. Kalet, immediately sensing the parallels between the emerging pandemic and the attack on the World Trade Center, shared her memories of 9/11 as a parent of young children and junior faculty member at New York University.

On the morning of September 11, 2001, I dropped my daughter with our babysitter and my son at his second grade class. The sun was shining and the air was clear as I took the stairs down to the New York City subway platform and headed to work at the medical school. When I emerged from the subway, I noticed people on the street, who normally would be rushing off to work, congregating in small groups or anxiously talking on their phones. I passed a television and saw, for the first time, The Twin Towers with gray smoke streaming from their midsections.

The rest of that day was not a blur. Every minute is burned into my memory. They still replay.

Within twenty-four hours, I was on a team of physicians, each of us with prior training in group facilitation, deployed to provide psychosocial support for the residents who waited anxiously for the wave of very sick and gravely injured patients that never materialized.

Today, physicians, nurses, healthcare workers, and public health administrators around the world are faced with dramatic surges of very ill patients, limited resources, and difficult ethical decisions. This time, the surge will surely come. We are them. They are us.

Now, we wait. What I have learned is that how we respond to emergencies matters.

Where is my Tool Belt?
Adapting to the New Realities

Wendy Peltier, MD

Dr. Peltier, who was Chief of the Froedtert & MCW Palliative Care Section, lamented that many of the traditional techniques of palliative and hospice care were impossible when caregivers were fully wrapped in PPE and families were kept from the bedside.

In normal times, palliative care team members work up close with patients and families, offering clinical expertise, goal discernment, and support at a patient's most challenging life transition. Our "tools" include our hands-on clinical expertise, where we touch and listen to our patients to diagnose and treat symptoms. We focus intently on empathic communication—both verbal and non-verbal—to provide support and to encourage understanding. We sit shoulder-to-shoulder with families, linking them to nursing, spiritual, community, and child life support services. We share long intervals of silence in close proximity, permitting time for everyone to process difficult news while allowing for deep-seated emotions to emerge. We gather weekly for our interdisciplinary team conferences to debrief cases and develop care strategies as a group. Our tool belts include an abundance of team approaches that enable us to manage conflict, share coping strategies, engage in corridor conversations, facilitate group meetings, and give hugs. It is how we work.

Isolation has a profound impact on end-of-life care and planning

As the risks of COVID-19 became evident, our hospital changed overnight. Patients facing this frightening, new disease with uncertain outcomes needed more support than ever, but the dangers of viral infection forced us to prohibit our dying patients from having visitors. We limited our own contact with patients to conserve personal protective equipment and held our team meetings by conference call. Dynamic changes evolved, such that we wore masks and eye protection even for patients without the virus. We sought ways to link to families remotely for goal setting. Our team, like so many others, worked in scrubs that we removed and washed as soon as we got home. Any time we spent working from home was filled with virtual meetings and constant worry of what was to come. This was a time to pull out all our tools, but our tool belts were out of reach.

Things have evolved

As our hospital activated video visits and encouraged connecting patients to their families via iPads, we learned the power of these connections, although we also witnessed the shock families experienced when finally seeing a sick loved one for the first time in days or weeks. Emotions ran very high, and we wished we could place a hand on a shoulder or even assure families that the visiting rules would soon be lifted.

Our team is not alone. We are partnering with other palliative care providers locally and nationally to develop and implement new strategies. It has been daunting, yet inspiring. Everyone misses the close contact upon which we depend. We have partnered with hospital administration and nursing leadership to develop visitation protocols that accommodate end-of-life visitors, albeit far from our "normal."

End-of-life care is best when it is low-tech and high-touch

Everything came into focus for me recently when the mother of one of my colleagues from work was admitted to our unit, nearing the end of her life. Caring for a relative of one of our own amplified our desire to make the patient's and family's last moments as fulfilling as possible. Despite the limitations, we created meaningful experiences. Since my colleague's loved one did not have the virus, she was able to spend time with her mother, a gift that our other patients are not able to share. She had the technology resources and creativity to connect her mother to all of the grandchildren via Facetime. A few cherished items from home warmed the room. Relatives were able to safely travel from out of state for support.

As I sat in her room, hearing stories of her mother and family in happier times, I felt a sense of grace and peace despite my mask and goggles. I realized how much I have missed these bedside conversations and long for the day when the COVID-19 danger has passed.

We who practice palliative care and hospice are commonly asked, "How can you do this work, day in and day out, and stay afloat?" My response is often that I can't imagine *not* doing this job and have always viewed it a special privilege to provide guidance and comfort at such a sacred time. Although we often deal with intense emotions, we also witness true love within families, facilitate ways to stay in the moment, and celebrate life even as death approaches. This present challenge has only intensified the value and richness of what we do.

Practicing in the COVID-19 pandemic has included new work rules, PPE, computer meetings, and a longing for the day when things approach normal again. We have developed a new appreciation for our old high-touch, up close, sitting together toolbelts. The day we get to strap them on again can't come soon enough.

Three Questions for a Frontline Worker Who Works with the Dying and the Bereaved

Angela Polcyn, MS

Ms. Polcyn, a Bereavement Coordinator at Froedtert Hospital, responded to questions about how the pandemic changed her work yet how important it was to stay the course. As a thanatologist, she focuses on the needs of the terminally ill and their families.

Transformational Times:
What has surprised you most about responding to the COVID-19 outbreak?

Angela Polcyn: One of the most surprising experiences of finding myself in the midst of the COVID-19 crisis is how my relationships with my colleagues have changed. We are in uncharted water and finding out how to swim together. My conversations have more grit and honesty. I am experiencing my own personal and professional vulnerabilities as well as those of every single person working in healthcare right now. We have found the willingness and the need to give a voice to our collective experience; to honor the burden of our responsibility, the uncertainty of the future, and the pain of our grief.

With this experience, every day is a lesson in resilience. We are having to renegotiate our sense of control, identity, and how we find meaning both professionally and personally, and we are building relationships and levels of trust with our colleagues that will forever connect us.

Transformational Times:
What have you found that families need most?

Angela Polcyn: As a thanatologist, my primary goal is to support the bereaved. Most normative grief trajectories include accepting the reality of a loved one's death and the process of restoring a sense of well-being. The current situation we are in has derailed this process. Most of the bereaved families I have spoken with are still in a state of shock and numbness, and rightly so. As the days and weeks go on, and we continue to be isolated and cut off from our support systems, death rituals, cultural connections, and our ability to collectively grieve, our responses and experiences will be delayed.

We are a community in the center of crisis, and our focus is on practical concerns. This is okay. Just because so many of the bereaved are not yet able to face their grief and sit with it, that does not mean there is something wrong. Delayed grief can be an adaptive response. Families are waiting to touch the rawness of their grief until they are able to gather, mourn, support one another, and take that first step toward restoring a sense of well-being. They are graciously making peace with a situation they cannot change. This gives me hope.

Transformational Times:
What advice can you share for dealing with grief?

Angela Polcyn: The experience of grief is already isolating, and it cuts us off from friends and family. Not only this, but as healthcare professionals, we also have an added sense of responsibility and purpose. It is okay to acknowledge your suffering as a healthcare professional right now. Fight the urge to minimize your pain. You have every right to it.

If you find this difficult to do, then view your suffering in the context of the larger perspective, but do not lessen its validity. See it for what it is and give yourself permission to honor your pain and experience, and open up the space for self-compassion. List out the things you have lost; name them, speak them out loud.

Self-compassion is about attending and befriending our struggles, making a place for them in our narrative. Finding truth in our suffering, making a place for it, and holding space for others who are suffering. This is the self-compassion we need right now.

The Emotional Toll of Being a Healthcare Provider During a Global Pandemic

Paul A. Bergl, MD

Dr. Bergl, a physician who spent the early months working in the Intensive Care Unit, labored to care for the sick and dying. A few months after the pandemic hit, he looked back to catalogue the emotional rollercoaster on which he had ridden.

In this loosely chronological reflection, I do not assume that I have captured the sentiments of many of my colleagues; instead, I only offer my own. And I hope that I have made evident my sincere sympathy for those suffering greatly from the fallout of COVID-19 and my perpetual gratitude for those working even harder than I am.

Naivete

I remember my first reaction to COVID-19 in February 2020 was blithe naivete. Skeptical of media hysteria, I encouraged friends and families to keep on with their daily lives. "You are far more likely to die from a bolt of lightning than a novel virus spreading overseas."

Exhilaration, sorrow, and elation

After coming to my senses as SARS-CoV-2 spread among our neighbors, I next experienced exhilaration. Here was my moment to fulfill the great dreams I had as a twenty-something applying to medical school: To save lives! To be part of living history! To serve on the front lines of a crisis! Rapidly elevated to hero status, I dutifully reported to my clinical roles and spent most waking hours helping my colleagues prepare for Armageddon. We developed protocols. We debated how we would allocate scarce resources. We strategized about how to save our medical students' education. Despite long hours in the ICU and countless email exchanges and Zoom meetings outside of my clinical work, I was indefatigable.

Of course, incredible sorrow interspersed these periods of elation. I witnessed patients succumbing to COVID-19 in airtight rooms, devoid of any symbol that they indeed were a person. No family. No photos of loved ones. No spiritual guides. No favorite sweatshirt. Who wouldn't cry after holding the phone to a dying octogenarian's ear while her family pleaded with an unyielding fate?

Guilt and anger

Soon, guilt settled in. Guilt that I had regular opportunities to see real actual live people while millions of lonely people huddled indoors comforted, at best, by faces on screens and, at worst, discomforted by total solitude. I dutifully reported to a job in which solidarity was high; we had a shared sense of purpose in a fight against a new enemy. Why should I have any sense of grief when so many collected unemployment? Or experience the exasperation of witnessing racial injustices on two fronts? Or suffer through the grief of losing a loved one to a crisis partly of our own society's making?

Then came a rising and ultimately unmitigated anger. My fellow citizens began flouting social distancing. My leaders began politicizing every part of the fight. Millions assumed that because most cases were mild that the entire thing had been blown out of proportion. These attitudes depreciated not only the work my colleagues and I were doing in the ICU every day, but also the efforts of our greater scientific, medical, and public health communities. Yes, I am still pretty pissed off.

Malaise

For two weeks in August 2020, I suffered a profound malaise, and was diagnosed with a so-called "mild case" of COVID-19. It sapped not only my energy and sense of smell, but also my optimism that we were turning the corner on a crisis. To add insult to injury, I believe I contracted the virus while performing a bedside procedure that conflicted with my own values, but a procedure that I was ethically obligated to provide nonetheless, at least within the framework of how we provide healthcare in America.

Now, as cases surge to their highest levels, I can see the lassitude that heralds burnout on my own face and those around me. I try to remind myself every day that I am privileged. And I am. I try to ignore the outside noise when I am at the bedside. "Remember, Paul, your obligations are to this patient, this human being, and you need to be the best damn doctor you can be right now."

Sadly, there are few outlets to recharge from exhaustion these days. And after all, depersonalization is probably adaptive, right?

No Words Can Describe the Experience of Caring for COVID-19 Patients in the Community

Michelle Minikel, MD

Dr. Minikel, a primary care physician with Bellin Health in Green Bay, WI, worked in an early COVID-19 hotbed. In this essay, she shared the emotional toll of caring for people in a community where her underserved patients bore a disproportionate burden of the pandemic.

Over the past few months, I have been interviewed, served on a panel discussion, given a lecture, and written an essay about what it was like to care for a disadvantaged population during a major COVID-19 outbreak in Green Bay. I said yes to these opportunities, but it was hard. I don't usually feel up to the task. I don't know if I can really put to words what this pandemic has been like.

How can I convey the frustration . . .

. . . of seeing the first positive SARS-CoV-2 test result of a patient of mine who works at a meat packing plant? The very same patient who had asked me a couple of weeks prior for an excuse from work due to her high-risk health conditions? She later informed me that her request to be excused from work was denied.

. . . of having toured the plant and seen the working environment. How can I ever describe what it was like to know, just know, that COVID-19 was going to tear through that plant like a tornado? It wasn't a surprise; we had already seen it happen in multiple similar workplaces. But the public health department was powerless to close the plant. I will never know if there is more that I could have done to close it, even if for just a couple of weeks. A couple of weeks that could have perhaps saved a couple of lives.

How can I convey the heartache . . .

. . . of what it was like to see a once-hospitalized COVID-19 survivor, back to see me in the clinic, whose husband didn't make it, who didn't survive the infection she brought home from work?

. . . of seeing the patient who also blew whistles at her meat packing plant in early March 2020 and whose requests to wear a mask were denied? "We matter less to them than the cows," she told me.

. . . of what it was like to see two of my pediatric patients in clinic and finally meet their premature newborn baby sister, taken from her mom's womb as she died at age thirty of COVID-19?

How can I convey the anger . . .

. . . that the meat packing plants wouldn't close down and instead let the fire rage for days, stoked with bonuses for the employees who did not miss work? Are our hamburgers really that essential?

. . . of hearing people decry the springtime 2020 Green Bay outbreak as stemming from a lack of education among the Hispanics? Day after day in the clinic, I heard about their fears of continuing to work and the sacrifices they were making to protect themselves, and answered their questions about how to best prevent the virus. All while watching hydroxychloroquine be given to them in the hospital, in many cases, even weeks after the CDC stopped recommending it.

. . . of watching people in Green Bay, even now, shop without masks and continue to go out to restaurants and bars, while our children aren't able to attend school?

No words can describe this experience.

COVID-19 and Grief

Cassie Ferguson, MD

Dr. Catherine (Cassie) Ferguson, an Associate Professor of Pediatrics (Emergency Medicine) at MCW, runs a wellness course for medical students. In this essay, created early in the pandemic, she shared how her professional and personal life were being affected.

This week I came across a Facebook post written by a friend from junior high school. She shared an article published in the *Harvard Business Review* written by Scott Berinato entitled "That Discomfort You're Feeling is Grief." (3/23/2020). The article features an interview with Dr. David Kessler, a well-known bioethicist and expert on grief, loss, death, and dying. In the interview, Kessler confirmed that the conditions are ripe for people to be grieving. "We feel the world has changed," he says, "and it has. We know this is temporary, but it doesn't feel that way, and we realize things will be different."

Grief.

That word resonated right away with me. *I am grieving,* I realized. *That is what this feeling is.*

I grieve for the dead as a result of this virus and for the thousands to come. I grieve for my colleagues here and abroad who feel the weight of this pandemic on their shoulders, and for those who have lost their lives in service of their profession. I grieve for people who have lost their jobs, for people who own small businesses, for people with mental illness, and for people who live in nursing homes. I grieve for those who live with an abuser. I grieve for our learners who want to help and have been told no, and for those who will miss major milestones in their education. I grieve for my grandmother who died earlier this month and whose memorial service has been postponed indefinitely.

Maybe you have struggled with grief in the past, as well. You may feel, as I do, that the coping mechanisms that have worked before suddenly seem inadequate in the face of a global pandemic.

Kessler recommends that those who are working through grief keep trying. *"There is something powerful about naming this as grief,"* he says. *"It helps us feel what's inside of us. So many have told me in the past week, 'I'm telling my coworkers I'm having a hard time,' or 'I cried last night.' When you name it, you feel it and it moves through you. Emotions need motion. It's important we acknowledge what we go through...We tell ourselves things like, 'I feel sad, but I shouldn't feel that, and other people have it worse.' We can—we should—stop at the first feeling. 'I feel sad. Let me go for five minutes to feel sad.' Your work is to feel your sadness and fear and anger whether or not someone else is feeling something."*

He goes on to say, *"Fighting it doesn't help because your body is producing the feeling. If we allow the feelings to happen, they'll happen in an orderly way, and it empowers us."*

I recognize that all of this takes an enormous amount of courage, particularly for those of us who have experienced catastrophic grief in our past. Yet, what I've found is that in recognizing and turning towards grief, it feels somehow as if I am honoring all those that I grieve for.

Keep reaching out. Love and light to all of you.

Responding to the Pandemic: Practical Wisdom in Action

Adina Kalet, MD MPH

Very early in the pandemic, when COVID-19 cases were rapidly rising in New York City, Dr. Kalet wrote about how the pandemic-induced disruption of the medical system affected what should have been a simple and treatable illness.

This past Sunday, Fred (not his real name) became acutely disoriented, physically agitated, and distressed, likely as a consequence of another antibiotic-resistant urinary tract infection. Over the course of his eighty-nine years, Fred has been an accomplished novelist, creator of children's books, a Korean War veteran, a rabid baseball fan, and a chocoholic. The past couple of years, though, have brought changes for Fred and his wife, Josephine. As his memory faded, they have been increasingly confined to their New York City apartment. That said, they have continued to enjoy their time together, often sharing good food, classic movies, and reruns of old baseball games.

Their apartment is just a few blocks from the public hospital, his medical home. Fred is smitten with his brilliant and caring geriatrician, Dr. Lee. Under normal circumstances, when he gets sick, Fred and Josephine call her and she meets them in the emergency room for lab tests, antibiotics, and a liter or two of IV fluids. A visiting nurse stops by the apartment a couple of days later to provide an assessment and collect a urine sample. This has happened before and worked well.

But these are not normal times in New York City.

The weekend Fred fell ill, physicians and nurses' phones were being diverted to call centers, and all of the emergency rooms were jammed. There weren't enough healthy visiting nurses to cover homecare duties. A trip to the ER would have meant a long, lonely wait for Fred, separation from Josephine, and exposure to people with COVID-19. If Fred had been septic, he would have been hospitalized. If his breathing deteriorated, the treating team would have had to decide whether to intubate him and place him on a ventilator, but during a citywide scarcity of ventilators, supporting Fred in an ICU might not have been a priority. The faculty and residents would have then faced a difficult choice: *Under what circumstances should they withhold care from one human being to ensure it is available for another? What criteria do they use?*

Decisions regarding advanced support hinge on the likelihood of recovery, but these criteria can be tricky to apply to individuals. While no one wants to discriminate based entirely on age, mental capacity, or physician ability—any more than anyone would ever condone making these decisions based on socioeconomic status, profession, or skin color—our socialization influences us unconsciously. Hospital systems and states provide guidance on how and when to ration ventilators and ICU beds, but ultimately every choice requires a physician to exercise extraordinary self-awareness, mustering courage and judgement in the face of uncertainty.

In the Kern Institute, we emphasize the integration of the competency, capacity, character strength, and professional identity needed to be a good doctor. This Practical Wisdom—the ability to do the right thing at the right time for the right reasons—is starkly evident during public health catastrophes like the COVID-19 pandemic, but should always be a core aspiration for every good physician.

Luckily, years before COVID-19, Fred and Dr. Lee had discussed his wishes to avoid hospitals at the end of life. Once Josephine and the family contacted her, she helped arrange for home hospice. Fred stayed in his apartment and was provided with sedatives and reassurance. Dr. Lee did this even as she was being redeployed away from her primary care practice in order to back up her exhausted colleagues at the hospital.

Before long, Dr. Lee was caring for the sickest of the sick in high-intensity settings where she rarely worked. She worried that she might soon be in over her head. She trusted, though, that her colleagues and the nurses would help. She gathered her courage, humility, and practical wisdom, and she headed to the hospital.

Make it to the Mat: Perseverance and Adversity When a Parent is in the Hospital with COVID-19

Katie Recka, MD

*Katherine (Katie) Recka, MD, an Assistant Professor
of Medicine (Geriatric and Palliative Care) at MCW,
practices palliative care. In the early days of the pandemic,
her family's inability to visit her critically ill father made
her worry about how they would help him recover.*

It was March 31, 2020. I was happily isolated in my VA office, attending a WebEx meeting. My phone vibrated. It was Mom. Probably a misdial. She only calls in emergencies. Couldn't she just text?

I was already grabbing my coat and keys before the voicemail was done. Something was wrong. It was Dad. Stomach pain, coded in the emergency room, now in the ICU. Or was it surgery?

That night we huddled together in my childhood home, just two blocks from the hospital in Green Bay. We were so close to him, but we may as well have all been in Texas for the good it did us. All we could do was stare at the pictures flashing by on the television and wait for the calls. It was Netflix, and the show was an episode of the docuseries, *Cheer*, and my father was dying.

He's out of surgery.

He's on three pressors.

This doesn't look good.

We have certain visitor exceptions; would one of you like to visit?

All with the sunny inanity of the television in the background, its face-to face intensity now archaic. There are no masks in the cheerleader pyramid, no social distancing.

Now I was the one who was spinning and disoriented. My father didn't have COVID-19, but the presence of the virus in the community would keep all of us out of the hospital, my second home. Now I was (*gasp—double flip—will she make it?*) a patient's family member, not a doctor. I wasn't an insider. I was a helpless daughter, the annoying daughter who kept calling, the daughter born forty years ago in the same building where Dad was intubated, sedated, alone.

We build our own pyramids within our health systems, vibrant and wholesome when they work well, but precarious when they don't. The days ticked by. At first, Dad was too delirious to use the phone in the ICU. He didn't remember why he was there, but he was desperate to get out. Then he was in acute care, and he was terrified knowing he might never get back to his family and to his home that was so close, we were almost visible from the window of his room. Finally, he was in sub-acute rehab that we promised would be better but wasn't. Each step was filled with well-meaning experts who couldn't accommodate the one thing my father needed, the reassuring voice of a loved one unfiltered by electronics.

We built layers of help. Home care promised light and fresh air, but with face masks and eye shields, would we even recognize his home nurse if we saw him in the grocery store? The gear protected everyone from an invisible virus but isolated us. How do you bond with the strangers in your own home when they are faceless?

The whole goal in *Cheer* is to "make it to the mat." The athletes practice until they collapse. They run, jump, and flip to the finals despite both physical and spiritual injuries. We watched Dad move painfully from bed to chair. Then he could walk, then take on stairs. A high-five from everyone when he ate at the kitchen table and support when he kept his game face on during the complicated reality of closing the law office he had opened ten years before I was born.

I can and will slip back into my comfortable role, but what do I do now as an insider? The provider with a new normal? We keep going until we get it right. Our well-trodden path to the conference room is now the well-worn keyboard on our computer. It's WebEx, Zoom, Skype, FaceTime, Facebook, Instagram, text, and phone.

We attack this new normal like athletes do. We need to do it again, and do it again, and do it again so that constantly making connections becomes our normal. We nail that mental backflip until we believe that sheltering apart is sheltering together. If we don't believe that masks and eye shields and gloves facilitate contact instead of separate, what patient is going to believe us when we look through a layer of scratched Lexan and say things we don't believe in ourselves?

Keep going. Do it again. Make it to the finals. Somewhere, there is another father coding and another family out there spinning and disoriented. We need to be there to catch them. We need to stick this landing hard and leave it all on the mat.

Building Trust with the Underserved Community During a Pandemic

Christopher Davis, MD, MPH

Christopher Davis, MD, MPH, Assistant Professor of Surgery (Trauma and Acute Care Surgery), works in community outreach. In this essay early in the pandemic, he highlighted how the pandemic was disproportionately affecting communities of color and how the institution was called to respond.

COVID-19, like so many other diseases, strikes communities of color disproportionately. As of April 1, 2020 most of Milwaukee's COVID-19 cases and deaths have been in the African-American community.

Here's a frightening, real-life illustration: On February 29, 2020, about two hundred friends and relatives attended the funeral of Andrew Jerome Mitchell, a retired janitor, in the small, rural, poor, underserved community of Albany,

Georgia. It was one of two funerals held at the same chapel over the course of a few days. Andrew came from a large family, and the room overflowed. The mourners shared a potluck and told stories. No one was known to be ill at the time. After the funeral, everyone went their separate ways. In the ensuing weeks, dozens of the mourners—and then their contacts—became ill. Over the past four weeks, over six hundred people eventually contracted COVID-19, including six of Andrew's siblings. The local hospital was overwhelmed. So far, at least twenty-four have died, including Andrew's fifty-one-year-old great-niece. The death rate per capita is nearly that of Wuhan at the height of the outbreak.

Ninety percent of the victims in Albany were African-American.

Albany offers a cautionary tale for Milwaukee. A 2019 Wisconsin Collaborative for Healthcare Quality report confirms that Milwuakee's lowest socioeconomic communities (primarily African-American and Latinx) have measurably worse levels of blood pressure control, blood sugar control, immunization rates, appropriate heart disease management, and life expectancy than whites. So when a disease like COVID-19 strikes hardest at individuals who have "preexisting conditions," communities of color are disproportionately affected.

As a society and a community, we expect everyone to work to "flatten the COVID-19 curve." We recognize, though, that the vulnerable are the least prepared to practice social distancing, since they disproportionately work in service and personal care industries and fulfill "essential" functions. Many cannot stay home for weeks since they are one paycheck away from homelessness. These people (people!) suffer the centuries-old consequences of health and educational inequities and are separated from the rest of society by income disparities, embedded racism, housing insecurity, nutritional deserts, inadequate transportation, low literacy rates, and a lack of adequate health insurance.

MCW depends on—and benefits from—its ties to the community. We know people are fearful and grieving. They thirst for clear, evidence-based information to keep themselves and their loved ones healthy and alive. They need supplies and accompaniment. Milwaukee's underserved deserve true leadership and, since the bonds of trust between the underserved community and medicine are fragile, essential leadership must come from within the community itself. To this end, many within MCW are working to support our underserved communities and their leaders.

As an organization, we pledge to communicate essential, factual, timely, and community-appropriate information and to leverage our strengths to provide meaningful resources.

It is not a question of whether we will serve either our community or serve our front-line healthcare workers. Rather, the answer is "yes and." Doing so is a matter of justice as we treat others not only fairly, but also by accounting for different levels of need. We are marshalling medical students and non-front-line MCW community members to serve the underserved community by providing protective masks and offering education. We hope that by "showing up," we play a small role in healing generations of well-deserved mistrust between the African-American and Latinx communities and medicine.

Our missions are to help every member of the community through the COVID-19 pandemic, to not overlook the forgotten, and to build ties that will solidify trust on which our common future depends.

Embracing the "New Normal," and Who Gets to be a Physician

Adina Kalet, MD MPH

Dr. Kalet, in an essay published when it was becoming clear that things would not be going back to normal anytime soon, wrote about how the application process would likely change for both medical school and residency positions. She suggested that we learn from this opportunity and think about what we might want to adopt for the future.

It is an open secret that it is far harder to get into medical school than to stay in. Only 41% of applicants to medical school are accepted in any given year, while medical school graduation rates are over 95% within six years of acceptance, and 96% of graduates go on to match into a residency training program. It is possible, however, that COVID-19 might change all of that.

Normally, we would be preparing for interview season now

For decades, fall meant the arrival of groups of twenty-somethings, wearing conservative blue suits and pulling rolling suitcases, marching through hospital lobbies and medical school hallways all over the US. These gaggles were invariably trailing either a medical student guide or a bedraggled but authoritative chief resident in a well-worn white coat with clogs peeking out from under scrub pants. It's interview season, when over 53,000 medical school applicants and 35,000 residency applicants go to great effort and expense, crisscrossing the United States, to chase their dreams.

As they peer into classrooms, learn about schedules, and share lunch with faculty and other applicants, each one hopes to experience that "gut feeling" about the "fit" between themselves and the institution. Meanwhile, admissions deans and residency program directors, after sifting through digital mountains of applicant data to select interview candidates, hope to end the day with a sense of who best fits with their schools and programs. While this seems like a sacred rite of passage, it will not be for the foreseeable future.

COVID-19's impact on residency applicants

The Residency Match will change for 2020-2021. On May 11, 2020, the Coalition for Physician Accountability—a cross-institutional group of national medical education organizations—released recommendations to alter "Current

Practices of Student Movement Across Institutions for the Class of 2021" as follows:

- Students will not be able to do away elective rotations.
- All interviews will be conducted virtually.
- The Electronic Residency Application Service® (ERAS®) residency match timeline will be pushed back to allow students to complete their graduation requirements.

The first two, particularly, will fundamentally change the process of residency selection for the coming year. Medical students will be unable to "audition" at their favorite institutions. Residency programs will be unable to glean the intangibles that crop up during day-long, on-site interviews. For the upcoming year, at least, the transition between medical school and residency will change.

COVID-19's impact on medical school applicants

Medical school applicants, similarly, face substantial changes. Interviews and school visits will almost certainly be virtual. MCAT test dates have been canceled from March through May 2020, and more dates will be canceled, if necessary. There is no precedent. We have no idea how this will impact how we decide who gets into the long pipeline toward becoming a practicing physician.

The impacts will be both bad and good

Except for the rare, outstanding, top-tier applicant who needs no interview, most students and residents have educational metrics in the middle of the pack. While they have the most to gain by interviewing well, they will have to be prepared to accept the choice they are offered. This reality will test their humility, tolerance of ambiguity, and integrity. Despite their personal ambitions, this occasion to make the absolute best of their "good enough" option will demonstrate character traits that are critical components of what it means to be a physician.

There will also be some immediate benefits, however. Not having to travel for interviews will save applicants, in aggregate, at least $800,000,000. This represents about $10,000 per applicant, an amount that most do not have and, therefore, would have added to their educational indebtedness. The applicants who stay closer to home will have hidden benefits of lower housing and childcare costs. And, thanks to Zoom, maybe they purchase only a new sport coat or jacket rather than an entire suit.

Challenges to medical schools and residency programs

Without campus visits, our medical school and residency programs might find it more challenging to convince the best applicants that Milwaukee is a great place and that MCW offers a unique sense of "family." Although virtual interviews, done well, might provide unique affordances, we will likely miss the subtle clues that an otherwise excellent candidate would not be a good cultural fit with the school or program. We will have to create social connections between the current and potential future members of our community while presenting a realistic but optimistic view of what is to come.

While the greatest institutional cost associated with interviewing is for the salaries of people who organize and run the events, there will be savings when institutions and programs do not need to provide food and hotel rooms for interviewees. In addition, interview strategies such as Multiple Mini Interviews, which better predict long-term clinical competence than the usual interview approaches, may be more cost-effective and feasible using available technology.

What opportunities can we leverage?

All schools and residency programs are committed to increasing diversity in students and trainees. Admissions practices and policies are the most powerful drivers to reduce unconscious bias and ensure that we attract physicians-to-be most likely to practice in underserved rural and urban settings. And while very complex, efforts to rebalance the proportions of specialists and primary care physicians to better meet the needs of the public while managing the quality and costs of care could be partly addressed through admissions policies. We have the potential to learn much in the next year.

Should we expand models of transition between educational phases? Thinking outside of the box

There are alternative models where students transition from one phase of education to another. For example, combined medical school/residency programs exist, such as the Education in Pediatrics across the Continuum (EPAC) program at the University of Minnesota and the three-year accelerated track of the NYU Grossman School of Medicine, where schools create efficient training continua focusing on educating the best physicians. We might also experiment with smoothing the UME-GME continuum. What if we accepted a certain number of students into medical school with a guaranteed residency spot at MCW?

Combined pre-medical/medical school programs have been around for decades. I entered the Sophie Davis School of Biomedical Science at the City College of New York (now the CUNY Medical School) straight out of high school, knowing that—if I worked hard—I would complete both my Bachelor's and MD degrees with fewer prerequisites, no MCAT, and a slimmed down medical school application process. I turned out okay, right? Countries with enviable healthcare systems have different approaches to applications and admissions, often awarding an MD or equivalent degree after six years of post-secondary education. There are many opportunities for meaningful innovation.

We must be kind . . .

COVID-19 will force medical schools and residency programs to explore new ways to screen, interview, and choose their next cohort of students and trainees. Schools and programs will make adjustments as they navigate these uncharted waters.

For applicants, the loss of the in-person interview means they will have difficulty developing their gut feelings about hidden curricula, faculty engagement, social cohesiveness, educational culture, and commitment to the surrounding populations and places. They will lack the opportunity to suss out the actual differences between the values a program espouses in its written materials and the actual lived experience of the program. Medical school and residency applicants, who often depend on online forums and comments, will find themselves bereft of meaningful advice. They will be forced to find their way through an opaque system for which there is no precedent.

This strange period in history offers us many opportunities to do our work better. I am certain that some of the changes that occur in the coming months will be valuable and enduring while others will not. As we move forward, though, let us remember that many of the applicants will feel adrift and scared. We can remind them that they are where they are because we believed in them, and we now reaffirm that we will support them as they move toward becoming caring, character-driving, and compassionate physicians.

Lessons on Resilience, Empathy, and Magic from *Life is Beautiful* & Roberto Benigni in the COVID-19 Era

Malika Siker, MD

Very early in the pandemic, Dr. Siker contributed this essay, drawing some parallels between the resiliency of her cancer patients and the resiliency of the protagonist in Life is Beautiful. *Even in a time of stress, "to laugh and to cry comes from the same point of the soul."*

In 1997, the Italian movie, *Life is Beautiful (La Vita è Bella)*, burst onto our cinema screens and became an international sensation. In this story, a Jewish father named Guido is imprisoned in a concentration camp with his son Giosuè and goes to absurd and humorous lengths to shield Giosuè from fully realizing the monstrous reality surrounding them. Roberto Benigni, who co-wrote, directed, and starred in the film, played this epic role with conviction, compassion, and comedy, challenging viewers to wonder how far they would go to spare their child from ugly truths. I recall Guido's charm, wit, and devastating wink, as well as how hard I worked to hold back tears as the credits rolled when first seeing the film as a college student. I am ashamed to admit that I was successful. Not a single tear fell.

The COVID-19 pandemic is not even remotely comparable to the horrors of Nazi Germany during World War II. There is no debate. Adolf Hitler and his accomplices murdered seventeen million innocent people in Europe as part of a pogrom of deliberate and systematic extermination over six years. However, I have found myself thinking of Guido's approach to life and have been inspired by his spirit as a physician, an educator, and a mother of young children navigating the COVID-19 crisis.

In *Life is Beautiful*, Guido's effort to protect his son and to fight for their survival brings meaning to his existence. In my cancer clinic, I come face-to-face with patients actively undergoing radiation therapy who are at high risk of COVID-19 complications. I spend my free time learning about COVID-19 so I can best protect and advocate for my patients to reduce their risk. It has been incredibly humbling to realize how little we understood when the virus reached our shores, and how much more we are going to need to learn to bring a decisive end to this current situation. The uncertainty and fear of the unknown are stressful, but I remember to stay *resilient* for my patients.

Realizing how lucky I am to have completed my own educational journey without facing a pandemic, I am driven to use my privilege to help our students succeed. As a health science educator, I am motivated to ensure that our learners continue to receive an outstanding educational experience. They must quickly adapt to an unprecedented landscape where there are no guidelines. They are banned from their classrooms and libraries while studying and taking exams in new environments. They are frustrated and worried about their futures. Some are being robbed of seminal life experiences like graduation ceremonies. When Giosuè's happy childhood is interrupted by war in *Life is Beautiful*, Guido feels *empathy* for him and seeks to preserve Giosuè's childhood during uncertain times.

As our family invents our own new traditions, I think about how Guido turns a dire situation into a comical child's game. After a day of work, I come home to a bustling household as a mother to young children. With children's activities and social events canceled, we spend more time together discovering and creating our own little enchanted world. We build forts, bake new delights, and indulge in spontaneous imaginative adventures together. We deal with schoolwork and household chores. Normalcy reigns while anxiety lurks. Our family has been given a beautiful gift. My children know there is an invisible enemy outside our walls, but we are determined to create a little *magic* for ourselves to get through these days.

Roberto Benigni has said, "to laugh and to cry comes from the same point of the soul, no? I'm a storyteller: the crux of the matter is to reach beauty, poetry, it doesn't matter if that is comedy or tragedy. They're the same if you reach the beauty." I reflect on his philosophy while juggling my roles as a physician, educator, and mother.

To persevere in the COVID-19 era, I look for moments of resilience, empathy, and a little bit of magic. When I am unsure of what to do next, I think of Guido and allow myself, finally, to cry.

A Virtual Night on Call: Preparing Students for Internship Despite the Pandemic

Adina Kalet, MD, MPH

Dr. Kalet, who for a number of years has organized a virtual Night on Call training for senior medical students who are weeks away from becoming interns, wrote about effectively adapting the program during the pandemic.

Ring! Ring!

The medical student clicks the mouse and looks at the face on her computer screen.

"This is Dr. M. You paged me?"

"Yes, Doctor, you're covering Mr. Jackson, right? He was ready to go home in the morning, but . . ."

So begins a three-and-a-half-hour immersive, simulated Night on Call we designed six years ago to assess each senior medical student's readiness for transition to internship as the final medical school clinical exam just before graduation. This year, for obvious reasons, the Night on Call exams are being conducted virtually and are much higher stakes, since students have been on a clinical pause and are unable to complete their graduation requirements in any other way.

On the computer screen are two colorfully outlined squares. In one, "Dr. M.," a soon-to-be graduate of MCW-Central Wisconsin, wears her white coat and is playing herself as a brand-new intern. In the other square is a nurse, "Mr. D.," who tells Dr. M. he arrived for his hospital shift to discover that Mr. Jackson in room 212 is having an unexpected, worrisome new problem. Dr. M. and Mr. D. discuss the case and agree to meet in Mr. Jackson's room to explore the clinical issues and make a plan.

A third square appears on the screen. It contains a middle-aged man wearing a hospital gown. Dr. M. introduces herself. *"Hi, Mr. Jackson, I am covering for Dr. Green. I hear you have a new problem."*

"No problem here! I'm just eager to go home tomorrow," answers Mr. Jackson.

And so it goes. Dr. M. cajoles Mr. Jackson to tell his story. She asks Mr. D. to share Mr. Jackson's lab results, EKG, and fluid intake and output (all done on the screen). Dr. M. lists the physical exam maneuvers she will conduct and why. Dr. M., Mr. D., and Mr. Jackson—who still insists on going home—agree on a plan. Dr. M. says goodbye, promises to return, switches screens, and writes a "cross-coverage note." She contacts the surgery attending on-call (whose role is played by her favorite clinical teacher and family physician) to present her findings and discuss the plan.

Dr. M. is called to see two more patients. Before the "simulated night" is over, she manages three patients and interacts on-screen with two more nurses, another attending physician, and a family member. She searches the internet for resources, interprets laboratory results and an EKG, writes clinical notes, and finally, once "morning" arrives, hands off the three patients to another clinician (played by another favorite clinical teacher).

She and two other students take deep breaths and undergo an online debriefing by a seasoned clinician. She thinks things went well, but she also realizes that there were gaps. She forgot to ask a couple of critical questions. She realizes that the other students were as anxious as she was. In a few days, she will receive an individualized, detailed report on her performance with prompts for self-assessment of her strengths and weaknesses and an opportunity to set learning goals. She is one step closer—and a bit more confident—as she prepares herself for internship.

Adapting the Night on Call to new institutions and a new reality

Colleagues at the NYU Grossman School of Medicine, The Texas Tech University Health Sciences Center School of Medicine, and MCW-Central Wisconsin have worked together over three time zones to develop and implement in-person Night on Call opportunities that assess the thirteen core Entrustable Professional Activities (EPAs) that the Association of American Medical Colleges (AAMC) has determined all graduates—regardless of future specialty—should be able to perform before entering residency. Night on Call is a feasible, reliable, and exciting way to assess whether near-medical school graduates are ready to assume their roles.

Therefore, when the AAMC recommended a pause in clinical rotations in mid-March 2020, the medical school deans approached the Liaison Committee on Medical Education (LCME) for permission to employ simulations and other virtual strategies to demonstrate students have achieved the core objectives and requirements for graduation. Our group sprang into action organizing, testing technology, and recruiting experienced Night on Call actors from around the country.

This week, twenty-five MCW-Central Wisconsin students participated in Night on Call. In mid-May, 2020, seventeen MCW-Green Bay students will go through the same experience.

Students have appreciated the opportunity to practice and get feedback. They tell us that the virtual structure, although artificial, feels authentic. Faculty members enjoy observing their students in action and are proud of how the students perform. One MCW-Central Wisconsin faculty member said that the day was a "moon shot."

"Nothing will be the same"

Our students are being launched into a rapidly changing healthcare landscape, and we must adapt as we prepare them. Telehealth will be front and center in their careers. Over the coming months, our graduates might find themselves trying out their history and physical skills while working in full personal protective equipment while they balance their fears with their compassion for the suffering of others. The decisions and challenges they face will be unprecedented. Even after the COVID-19 danger passes, nothing will be the same.

No one knows exactly what they will encounter. At the very least, by providing experiences like Night on Call, we help assure our near-graduates that they are ready to face the challenges offered by the next phase of their careers in medicine.

Graduation and Family

José Franco, MD

Dr. Franco, Interim Senior Associate Dean for Academic Affairs at MCW, wrote about how graduations are important to the families as they are to the people who walk across the stage, even in a time where ceremonies must be held virtually.

My daughter graduated from law school last weekend. Listening to her mom talk about mucus and her dad about poop at dinner had long soured her on a medical career. The ceremony was virtual and, I am sure, disappointing to many, but necessary during these challenging times. As the dean delivered his opening comments, I found myself becoming both proud and teary-eyed.

Graduations celebrate graduates, their numerous accomplishments, and the excitement of the next phase of a lifelong journey. Graduations, to me, have always been about family, their sacrifices, and the support they provide when things are going well but also when times are tough. As I watched my daughter receive her degree (we were not physically with her), my tears were replaced by a smile as memories of my own graduation surfaced.

My own medical school graduation

My graduation from MCW occurred in May 1990. My parents were coming to Milwaukee for the first time. I remember reassuring them about the excellent May weather and that light jackets would suffice. Of course, meteorology not being my forte (nor the weatherman's), it snowed eight inches two weeks prior.

Details of the graduation ceremony are sketchy after thirty years. The event was held on a weekend at the Milwaukee Exposition Convention Center and Arena (MECCA). This was the home of the Bucks, pre-Bradley Center and Fiserv Forum. Today, it is known as the UW-Milwaukee Panther Arena. I do not remember marching in nor marching out of the arena. I recall Leslie Mack, Registrar and Director of Admissions, reading my name as I was instructed to walk across the stage. I do not recall putting on my regalia, who the commencement speaker was (ironic, as I am now on the commencement committee and help select the annual speaker) nor, at the time, remembering the words of the Hippocratic Oath—words that would guide me through the years to cultivate caring and respect for my patients as I trained and practiced.

My parents were proud

What I do remember as if it were yesterday was how proud my parents were. As the immigrant son of a carpenter and seamstress, I was the first in the family to graduate college, and now I was a doctor. Throughout the ceremony, I focused on my parents in the audience. They had smiles throughout the duration. I almost wished they could have walked across the stage with me as I realized how much they had given up to make this day possible. I remember the embrace from my father and the hug from my mother once outside of the building. After the ceremony, we joked about how off-base the nuns and my elementary school teacher had been while I was growing up in Spain. The nuns had chased me off the convent grounds. In defense of both, I would occasionally forgo school and trespass on the convent grounds to scavenge giant bamboo because it made an excellent fishing pole.

I recall my parents reminding me to send them the formal graduation picture that was taken at the event (I only bought one and proudly sent it to them). My father passed away in 1997 and my mother in 2015. I think about them both every day. When I went through my mom's photo album after her death, my First Communion picture was on page one and my MCW graduation picture on page two. This fall, I will gather with my classmates as we celebrate our thirty-year reunion, whether in-person or virtually. My parents will be there with me, with the same smiles they had in May of 1990.

Over the next week, our soon-to-be graduates will be taking pictures on our three campuses. Many will have their parents and families with them. Graduating in this time of great uncertainty, they will not have the formal ceremony they so richly deserve. Nonetheless, our students will be smiling, as will their parents and families. Congratulate them both!

Every Virus Needs a Host and the Answer Lies Within Each of Us

Balaraman Kalyanaraman, PhD

As the pandemic raged on, Dr. Kalyanaraman, Professor of Biophysics at MCW, turned his practiced and acerbic eye on how the pandemic carries both echoes of the past and foreshadowings of the future.

I don't know about you, but the terms "social distancing," "self-quarantining," "asymptomatic," and "flattening the curve" were all new to me until just a few months ago! You are not alone if you're suffering from COVID-19 news fatigue and can't wait to have your "old and boring" life back ASAP.

It took me a while to figure out that social distancing is not the same as antisocial, and that self-quarantining is not a punishment. Apparently, social distancing existed in medieval times and was used to fight the bubonic plague.

Here is some historical "viral" news that may interest you.
Sir Isaac Newton (1643–1727)

Sir Isaac Newton (1643–1727), a transformative scholar, inventor, and writer, made all his discoveries in the fields of calculus, astronomy, optics, and gravitation while in isolation. In case you are new to social distancing history, here is my take.

Twenty-three-year-old Newton was studying at University of Cambridge in England in 1665, when London was hit with the Great Plague. The university temporarily closed, and Newton went to his family home in the countryside. Even then, the rate of infection was recognized to be much higher in densely populated cities than in the rural areas. He used his time off wisely and started to think boldly in isolation. No emails from or videoconferencing with professors! No social media! Newton spent a lot of time musing under an apple tree in the backyard, and legend has it that one afternoon he was bonked on the head by a falling apple. Rather than being miffed about it, he wondered why the apple fell straight rather than swerving, going up, or going sideways! Well, there you have it—the discovery of gravitational force. Newton also postulated the three laws of motion:

- Everybody remains in a state of rest or uniform motion unless acted upon by a net external force. How true! I saw it in a health club. Good motivational messaging! Now that I stopped going to the health club, I try to social distance with the refrigerator.

- The amount of acceleration of a body is proportional to the acting force and inversely proportional to the mass of the body; f = ma. I don't know why your car is so f@#*king damaged when you hit a deer at 70 mph.
- For every action, there is an equal but opposite reaction. Hmm, does this remind you of what is going on in Washington, D.C.?

Having worked out his theories on gravitation, calculus, and laws of motion, Newton returned to Cambridge after the plague subsided. He went from student to full professor in two years. By the way, the two years Newton spent in isolation and discovering new theories of nature are known as annus mirabilis or "remarkable years." Who knows? Some of our graduate students may realize 2020 was their annus mirabilis!

Sir William Shakespeare (1564–1616)

Many artists completed their classic works during isolation from a pandemic. Sir William Shakespeare (1564–1616) was one of them. Shakespeare was an actor, sharecropper and playwright. After an outbreak of bubonic plague, London's theatres were shut down and Shakespeare was out of a job! He decided to use his free time to write plays, including masterpieces like *King Lear* and *Macbeth*.

However, Shakespeare's most plague-inspired play was *Romeo and Juliet*, in which the plague and quarantine play a prominent role in the plot. Here are some *Romeo and Juliet* highlights and my thoughts on what Shakespeare can teach us all in the midst of COVID-19. Juliet and Romeo, from two feuding families in Verona, Italy, were in love but their families did not approve of their relationship. So, they secretly arranged to elope. In the meantime, Juliet's family decided she would marry someone else. Juliet's mentor had a counterplan to put her to sleep with a clever drug that would make her appear dead. A letter describing this plan was arranged to be delivered to Romeo. Spoiler alert: Romeo did not get the message because the messenger was quarantined and could not leave Verona due to the plague. You know the rest of the story.

So, what did Shakespeare teach us all that can be applied to COVID-19 and the 2020 presidential election? During a pandemic, mail delivery might be slowed down or even crippled, so people opting to vote absentee should do so in advance so their votes are delivered on time and uninterrupted.

2020 and COVID-19

Seriously, folks, we have a lot to be proud of. How can we forget the incredible sacrifices made by all the doctors, nurses, healthcare workers, scientists, firefighters, grocery store and delivery workers, IT professionals, and other essential workers that have kept us going? Recovered COVID-19 patients have given their plasma to COVID-19 ICU patients, saving their lives.

Automobile workers have repurposed their skills to make lifesaving ventilators. The list goes on. Stories of ordinary people doing extraordinary things abound in the time of COVID-19. An Arizona woman on an Indian reservation raised millions of dollars through GoFundMe to help the elderly and struggling families living without electricity or running water. These are our real heroes.

Years from now, 2020 will go down as our annus mirabilis

Every virus needs a host, but we don't have to be hospitable. At least part of the solution to keeping SARS-CoV-2 at bay is that we must continue doing the simple things to keep everyone safe—wearing masks, social distancing, washing our hands, sanitizing surfaces, and avoiding touching our faces. Let us remember our heroes and be grateful for all they have done for us.

Together, we will get through this.

Community Reflections: What is the Most Selfless Act You Have Seen This Week?

Rebecca Lundh, MD, an Assistant Professor of Family and Community Medicine, submitted this response:

My mother-in-law (elderly with multiple comorbidities) has told us that if she becomes seriously ill with COVID-19, she does not want to be placed on a ventilator. She wants to make sure younger people have access to this life-saving treatment.

Community Reflections: What Restrictions Have Affected You Most This Week?

Allison McLellan, MD, who, at the time, was a senior resident in Pediatrics, submitted this response:

I communicate via touch. A hand on the shoulder, a shoulder bump, a high-five; these are my social currency. My favorite transporter and I drop nonessential work to hug each other whenever possible. Today, it's different. We consider fist-bumping too much touch. We settle for a foot tap instead. He tells me, "You've got this, queen." This day, in particular, may be the least queen-like I've ever felt, unless queens thrive on social distancing and telemedicine. I suppose, on further reflection, that the queens of old used it to avoid lice and typhoid; I'll use it to protect my patients.

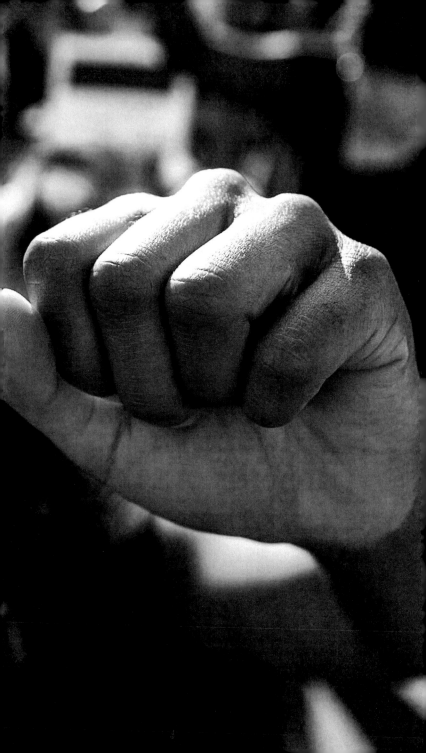

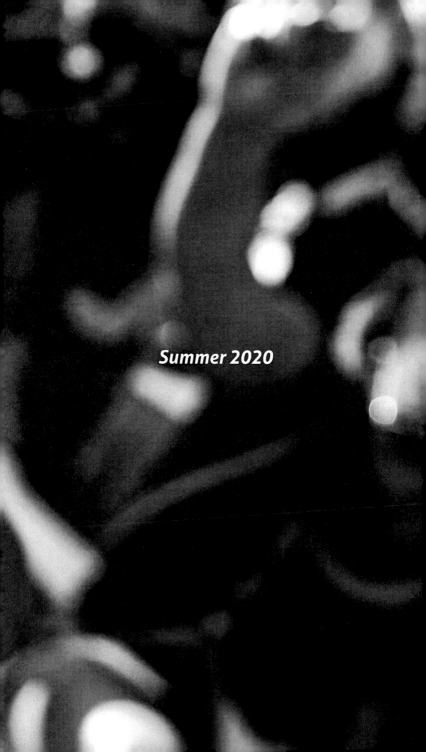

Summer 2020

Never Remain Silent: We Must Fight Systemic Racism as We Transform Medical Education

Adina Kalet, MD, MPH

Shortly after the killing of George Floyd on May 25, 2020, Dr. Kalet wrote about how the rapidly expanding societal awareness of systemic racism must also be addressed by medical educators. She emphasized that we need to stop making excuses for why our profession is not as diverse as it must be. "So, right now," she asked, "what do we do?"

"I swore never to be silent whenever and wherever human beings endure suffering and humiliation. We must take sides. Neutrality helps the oppressor, never the victim. Silence encourages the tormentor, never the tormented."
—Elie Wiesel

I have colleagues and friends who are afraid for their children. In the middle of a pandemic which is hitting communities of color—particularly African-American men and women—harder than other groups of Americans, professional colleagues in elite American academic institutions are not only worried about dying of the novel coronavirus, but they also fear being victims of violence because they are Black.

Early in March, when the CDC recommended that citizens use facial coverings to prevent the spread of SARS-CoV-2, some Black men feared they would risk being killed because they would be mistaken for criminals if they did so.

Horrific experiences are changing our narrative

The images are spellbinding: a police officer kneeling on George Floyd's neck as he begs for his mother, armed men in a pickup truck heading off Ahmaud Arbery as he jogs down a tree-lined suburban street, the snapshot of Breonna Taylor in her EMT uniform, smiling and holding a bouquet of flowers while the accompanying newspaper article documents how she was killed by police officers mistakenly serving a "no-knock warrant."

In New York City's Central Park, a Black man watching birds through binoculars asks a white woman to leash her dog. When she begins to rant at him, he records her on his cell phone. You see and hear the fear, terror, and outrage rising in her. She loses all reason, situational awareness, and compassion. Then you realize, *it is daylight in a well-traveled park and she has many options*. She could walk away, leash the dog, or continue to debate dog rights vs. bird rights. Instead, she chooses to call 9-1-1 and emphasize that she is being threatened by an "African American." What history and prejudices is she invoking? What is she thinking? *Is* she thinking?

These images and stories are shaking us from complacency, although our country has been accumulating irrefutable evidence of systemic racism over the past four hundred years. Are things different now? Can we do the anti-racism work needed to let justice roll down like water?

As a white woman, I search for hopeful signs in the aftermath of these events. There are some: social media carries videos of large, diverse crowds protesting peacefully across the country; news reports include images of police officers from San Jose and Queens "taking a knee" and walking arm in arm with anti-racism protesters; I hear people like Marine general and former Secretary of Defense James Mattis denounce the call for the use of the US military personnel against Americans on American soil.

So, what does all this have to do with transforming medical education? *Everything.* If physicians and scientists hope to improve the health and well-being of the populations for which they care and on whom they perform research, they must also address the root causes of racism.

Addressing the Weathering Phenomenon, Stereotype Threat, and the Minority Tax

Studies have long confirmed the strong association

between structural racism and poverty, and the literature confirms that health disparities are partly attributable to the cumulative exposures of the body to everyday forms of racism. Accumulated stress and epigenetic phenomena—i.e., the "allostatic load"—increase the risk of cancer, stroke, heart disease, and telomere shortening, all of which are associated with premature aging and death. This "weathering hypothesis" was first proposed in studies exploring why birth outcomes were abysmal for Black mothers and babies from all socioeconomic strata in the United States.

Racism causes unnecessary struggle. "Stereotype threat," first described by psychologist Claude Steele, is the predicament individuals face when they know the stereotypes others hold about them, and thus become anxious about confirming those stereotypes. Stereotype threat has been shown to contribute to long-standing racial and gender gaps in academic performance.

Medical school faculty members of color pay a significant "minority tax," because they are expected to provide disproportionately greater amounts of formal and informal mentoring of underrepresented minority (URM) students and institutional service on committees that seek racial diversity. Members of minority groups in medical schools risk being "tokenized," that is, being expected to represent and "explain" their group to well-meaning members of the majority group. Some medical schools are addressing these challenges head-on. Others are not.

Students and faculty of color in medical schools across the country experience unfair, unfriendly and, at times, frankly hostile environments. Medical school faculty of color are less likely to accomplish the usual academic milestones of promotion and tenure, less likely to obtain federal grants, and less likely to achieve pay equity.

As institutions and as fellow human beings, we must make sure we are fully aware and in control of our biases, embracing moral positions as allies to protect the lives of others. To be a masterful clinician, one must learn to recognize, and actively counteract, a host of predictable biases or prejudiced habits of mind. If we do not, unconscious biases, ignorance, and hijacking emotions will cloud our reasoning and behavior, leading to potentially fatal diagnostic and therapeutic mistakes. People will die.

So, right now, what do we do?

What does this have to do with transforming medical education? *Everything.*

Empathy, the key to therapeutic relationships, requires perspective-taking and a deep commitment to attend to others even when we are terrified, fatigued, or hungry. We can teach others how to do these things; however, without a strong, internalized medical professional identity and moral clarity, it might be impossible to enact this practical wisdom consistently and "do the right thing, at the right time, for the right reason."

We must explicitly educate ourselves and our community toward a mature identity where we consistently do right. To the white members of the community, it is our job to speak up and do the hard work of actively becoming allies. This requires courage and conversational skills which can be learned. This means facing what sociologist Robin DiAngelo has termed "white fragility" to describe the disbelieving defensiveness that white people exhibit particularly when they feel implicated in white supremacy. We have to be willing to have our feelings hurt, to engage in civil debate, and take action once we have some clarity.

We need to stop making excuses for why our profession is not as diverse as our population

Becoming diverse is the right thing to do. It will ensure our healthcare workforce can best serve everyone. This requires stable funding for programs to bring young people from underrepresented groups into the pipeline and creative strategies to keep them nearby for residency training. We must examine our assumptions about admission requirements, standardized testing, and academic potential. Recruiting a diverse student body and residency cohorts must go hand in hand with ensuring that learners from backgrounds underrepresented in medicine feel a sense of belonging once they matriculate.

My Black colleagues fear their sons and daughters are in an impossible and depressing situation. We must join together to keep their children safe and healthy. I, for one, am up for this challenge. I will vote, protest peacefully, have difficult conversations with my white colleagues and friends, and aspire to have a just society where all humans flourish.

The Disease of Racism

Sherréa Jones, PhD

A few days after George Floyd's killing, Dr. Jones, a current MCW-Milwaukee medical student, contributed this essay about racism.

Racism is a disease that inflicts every Black person in this country. We live with this disease our entire lives. There is no escaping it, overcoming it, or undoing it. The white people who infect us with this disease pretend to not know it is there despite perpetuating it, benefitting from it, and using it. Seeing the evidence of countless numbers of people suffering from it and the mounting dead bodies it has claimed that line the streets of every state in this nation is not enough for there to be any real attempt at addressing it.

The hard truth is, there is no cure for racism in this country, it was born this way. Every Black woman that gives birth in this country will knowingly pass this lifelong disease on to her child, although she tries to disguise it by giving her child a name that does not sound "too Black." The innocence of our childhood is stolen from us as we are forced to grow up in fear. Black people in this country are subjected to the damage of post-traumatic stress after witnessing our parents, children, and friends get slaughtered by this disease. Strangers that become permanent names in our minds are woven into our family trees by simply knowing that their treacherous death could have very well been our own. Black people suffer from an everlasting anxiety that no prescribed selective serotonin reuptake inhibitors (SSRIs) or serotonin-norepinephrine reuptake inhibitors (SNRIs) can control.

Racism was used to decorate this country with bold color lines, identical to the small, fancy blue street markers that highlight the sunny roads of Wauwatosa while the large green street signs of Milwaukee indicate, to those who are unfamiliar with the area, that you have traveled too far. The roots of systemic racism were used to decorate the halls of this institution with countless frames that hold pictures of white faces which serve as a constant reminder that I do not belong here. The ignorance of racism is being completely silent for almost a week on the most recent racist murder spree that stole the lives of Breonna Taylor, Ahmaud Arbery, and George Floyd. The acceptance of racism is knowing that the next class to matriculate here at MCW will not reflect the population that it will be called to serve. The burden of racism is knowing, wholeheartedly, that the string of letters that accompany my last name will never catapult me from the pressure of constantly having to prove my undeniable worth to this world.

As the mother of three Black sons in this country, I, too, made the conscious decision to bear children and pass down this disease to them. My soul aches for my children as I know that as much as I try to shield them from finding out they, too, are living with this disease, they will ultimately be given their diagnosis.

So, the next time, as a white person, you ask a Black person living in this country how we are doing, know that you have made the conscious choice to ignore the obvious agony of their disease and are forcing them to disguise it with a feeling that you are more comfortable acknowledging.

On Inclusion, Diversity, and Why Black Lives Matter Too: What Our MCW Community BLM Protests Mean to Our Colleagues of Color

Leroy J. Seymour, MD MS

Dr. Seymour, who was an Internal Medicine PGY1 at the time when he created this essay, wrote about the experience of watching Black Lives Matter protests on campus in the aftermath of the shooting of Jacob Blake in Kenosha, WI.

On Wednesday, September 2, 2020 at 5:11 pm, members of the Medical College of Wisconsin community held a Black Lives Matter protest to help shine a light on the frequent propensity for violence against people of color. This latest demonstration was one of hundreds of protests against police brutality and racial injustice that have been occurring in various cities, states, and countries, most recently triggered by the murder of George Floyd on May 25, 2020, in Minneapolis, MN. So many people have demonstrated peacefully and expressed their voices, all vying for the same dream Martin Luther King, Jr. expressed to the world. Almost every aspect of the world's population has provided an overwhelming outpouring of support of the Black Lives Matter movement, taking the baton and relaying the message that "Black Lives Matter, too" to widespread media coverage and the political stage.

MCW faculty, residents, and medical students alike raised their voices in support of the Black Lives Matter movement. This stance informed the world that MCW and the Froedtert Hospital community will not tolerate racism, and that racism itself is a pandemic that needs to be eradicated. The September 2 protest involved holding seven minutes of sustained silence, each minute representing every bullet aimed at the back of Jacob Blake, an African-American man returning to his vehicle, by Rusten Sheskey, a Kenosha, WI police officer. Mere seconds after violence left a man paralyzed, the world responded with outrage and exhaustion, yet another example of the unfair mistreatment of people of color when interacting with those with a perceived position of authority.

Many of us have protested these injustices before. I've protested it before. Our parents protested it before. Our grandparents protested it before. Our ancestors survived and protested it. I've stood face to face with the Ku Klux Klan, neo-Nazis, and individuals who have all decided that racial slurs and anger were the best response when asked why they hate people of color or different sexual orientation. Nobody should have to be afraid to walk outside or live in their own homes. People should not be judged by the color of their skin or their sexual orientation, but by the content of their character. People of every ethnicity, background, or creed should not have to be afraid for their lives when interacting with police. With the many communities, committees, social circles, and groups that I belong to, I can single-handedly attest to the importance of diversity, the inclusive nature of MCW, and why having people of varying backgrounds, experiences, and cultures is so critical to both the health of a community and a medicine brain trust.

As a new internal medicine resident and as an African American, I have witnessed firsthand the most beautiful sides of humanity, and the darkest corners of vitriol. I have cared for patients who have been incredibly appreciative and receptive of my presence, feeling more at ease with talking about their privileged information because I am a person of color. I have also had patients turn me away for the exact same reason.

When I wanted to become a physician, I made a lifelong commitment to improving and protecting my community. I've vowed to provide a safe haven for those without a voice, to be a vanguard in the face of hatred, to be the lighthouse in someone else's storm. But when it is you, your family, your friends, or your community who is being harmed, harassed, and violently mistreated, it takes that community to heal the hurt. It is hard to sustain a thriving and supportive community if that same community refuses to break bread with a particular subset of the population, even when everyone shares the same table.

I am proud to belong to a program and institution that takes a hard stance against institutionalized racism and is incrementally rolling out educational opportunities for those interested in, and in need of, anti-racism education. It is comforting to know that my colleagues and peers support the Black Lives Matter movement and understand the deeper inclusive meaning behind the statement. However, supporting the movement is only the first step of a marathon many have been running for years. With many cities in various countries now protesting the same cause, only time will tell if our collective voices have resonated, and what changes will result from our collective stance against institutionalized racism and racist ideology. Myself, my colleagues, and my peers at MCW have already decided which path we will walk, and that is hand in hand with our flourishing, diverse, and inclusive community.

Why We Need More Black Male Physicians

Victor Redmon, MD

Dr. Redmon, an MCW resident in Medicine and Pediatrics, wrote about two meaningful hospital encounters, and about how being a Black man shaped his development as a physician.

June 2016: A Black patient and his family

I am at the end of my third year in medical school and one week into my acting internship in the Veterans Affairs Medical Center Intensive Care Unit. The ICU fellow receives a call to transfer a cancer patient from the acute care floor to the ICU because of a concern he might be developing an overwhelming infection, or "sepsis." As the "intern" on the team, I eagerly accept the responsibility of taking the admission. I do a brief chart review and go to meet the patient and to gather more history. He is a Black male veteran, early fifties, frail and cachectic (characterized by physical wasting with loss of weight and muscle mass due to disease).

I introduce myself to him. "Hello, I am Victor Redmon, and I will be part of the ICU team caring for you downstairs." He looks me up and down. He responds, "You mean I'll actually have a Black doctor taking care of me? Well, that's all right," he says with a smile.

I meet various members of his family over the ensuing weeks, most of whom share the pride and adoration that they had a Black male caring for their loved one. I continue to take care of this patient for the remainder of the month.

He has a long and complicated ICU course, as he is dying and at the end stage of his cancer course. We conduct several family meetings to discuss goals of care and code status. The ICU attendings and fellows do an excellent job facilitating the meetings, and the family feels well informed. I am called to his bedside after one of these meetings. "I was told you had some questions for me," I say as I enter the room.

"Hi! We just wanted your medical opinion on what we discussed during the family meeting. What do you think we should do?"

Being a medical student at the time, I am completely caught off guard with such a heavy question. I respond with the same answers my attending and fellow provided earlier.

The family says, "Okay, thank you, Doctor. We just wanted to hear it from you because you are one of us." The patient passes away on my last day of the rotation.

April 2020: A Black hospital employee and his words

I am now a third-year resident serving as a senior resident for one of the inpatient pediatric teams. Like most days in the hospital, it has been very busy with admissions and duties on the medical floor. I have also not eaten breakfast or lunch and am starving by midday. I inform my interns that I am headed to the cafeteria for lunch and will be back soon. I head to the elevator and notice an environmental services worker waiting as well. He is a Black man, likely early to mid-twenties. The elevator arrives, and I gesture for the worker to get on first, since he has equipment to haul around. He says, "Thank you, Doc," and gets on the elevator.

I notice him staring at me and decide to make some small talk. I ask, "So how is the day going for you so far?"

He responds, "Not too bad, just another day. Are they treating you well here?"

I respond, "My work is busy, but all things considered I am very happy here."

He says, "Good, I am glad to hear it. Do you know how rare it is to see a Black male doctor?" The elevator dings, and the worker says to me as he exits, "I'll see you around, Doc. Keep up the good work. I am proud of you, I really am."

I respond, "Thank you, brother. I'll keep doing the best I can." The elevator doors close. I am alone.

July 2020: A reflection on what needs to change

I have had numerous interactions similar to what I've described above, but these two encounters I remember very vividly. As a medical student, I viewed these interactions as a source of pride and empowerment. My Black patients truly trusted me and related to me in a different way than they could with my non-Black colleagues. I have come to recognize the position I am in. No longer am I just any medical student, and no longer am I just another resident or trainee. I represent a source of pride and encouragement for the Black community. Truly, this is humbling. However, as I matriculate through my training, I ask myself more and more, "How and why?" Although I still feel a sense of pride and encouragement, I also have feelings of disappointment, sorrow, and isolation.

Through my experiences in training, I have become increasingly aware of the impact of underrepresented in medicine (URM) physicians when taking care of their representative patient populations. Of course, this is not a new concept. Many medical schools and graduate medical education programs, including MCW and Medical College of Wisconsin Affiliated Hospitals (MCWAH), have initiatives and policies in place that are centered around diversity. Yet, I believe that largely there has been little to no progress.

There have been many published studies that reflect the lack of progress with diversifying the racial-ethnic population of the medical schools and academic medical centers since the 1990s. Similarly, there are well-published studies illustrating the positive impact URM physicians can have with both the underserved population and their representative populations. URM physicians play a pivotal role in providing care where it is needed the most, which has been well documented and proven in several landmark studies. I believe there is a general intent to diversify our medical student and GME populations in order to be more representative of the people we are serving. Yet, I consistently see that diversity takes a clear back seat to academic achievement, which is defined by grades and standardized test scores.

My sentiments are not universal. There are many non-minority physicians who work extremely hard to provide excellent care to minority populations and underserved areas. There are even more people who work tirelessly on diversity and do not view diversity as an "extra," but rather as "necessary." I applaud and congratulate these people. I am blessed that I have been surrounded by individuals, many of whom are my colleagues and close friends, who truly feel that this is a critical area in medicine we need to improve upon.

I chose this topic to provide clarity and shed light on how URM physicians may feel day-to-day. Of course, I am not the sole voice for URM physicians—just a part of it—but I am not alone in my thoughts and experiences. I do not have a solution to the diversity dilemma, nor am I trying to give one. This is part of a larger socioeconomic discussion, which I believe traces back to our primary education system.

As Americans, we are at a truly unique and critical point in our history. We are in the middle of a global pandemic that has caused a significant economic and social strain on our society. Our society as whole is in the middle of political strife with the presidential election looming. We are in a unique era of social justice and potential social reform. I must say that I am worried about how racial relations may change as a result of what is currently happening in our country.

I am proud of the principles that my parents have taught and instilled in me. I am proud to be a Black American. I am proud to be a husband and father. I am proud of, and grateful for, the training I have received and the relationships I have built here at MCW and MCWAH. I am hopeful for the future.

Coronavirus and Inequity: Why Are We Shocked?

Christopher Davis, MD, MPH

In this call to action, Dr. Davis, a trauma surgeon, decried the suggestion that the pandemic was finally exposing inequities in society. "Those inequities were entirely clear decades and centuries ago."

———————————————————

These times bring what should be an unnecessary reminder of the need to care for one another as humans and the repercussions of not doing so. I remain dumbfounded at the suggestion that the coronavirus epidemic has "laid bare" the inequities in this country. Those inequities were entirely clear decades and centuries ago.

I'm not even sure what bothers me most these days. Is it that every day I'm on the Trauma Surgery Service, I take care of people who have been shot? Is it that 100,000 people have died in the four months since the first US

COVID-19 case was documented, while our federal response has been chaotic? Is it that my Venezuelan wife and children endure racist slurs and mistreatment nearly every single day for speaking Spanish and looking ever so slightly different, even though they are fluent in English and the American "culture"?

And, regarding culture, maybe what bothers me the most is the realization that some Americans simply do not value all human lives equally. This is downright embarrassing. It is stupid. It is ignorant. And it is wrong.

So, as COVID-19 cases mount in our Milwaukee, I would point out that the pandemic is not our only problem. In some neighborhoods, the life expectancy of African Americans is up to twenty years shorter than it is for people just miles away. As of May 31, 2020, sixty-two people in Milwaukee have died this year of homicide, up from just thirty-three by the same date last year. We have zip codes with some of the highest incarceration rates in the nation. And our infant mortality rates, a key benchmark of societal health, are consistently among the worst in the nation.

Our city, state, and nation are failing their citizens. It is at this point in history that, really, we have no choice but to do better. I pray we do, because the cost of human life that these United States have endured since before even the Revolution might finally be too much to bear.

The Gathering

David Nelson, PhD MS

Dr. Nelson, who works tirelessly for justice in our communities, wrote this essay about watching as people prepared for the opening of another day at the food pantry, noting that even hungry people were worried about gathering in groups.

The place will not be open for another four hours, and yet the people gather. There are three sets of numbers labeled 1-100 in colors of green, yellow, and blue. On a "normal" Saturday, several hundred would be served three to five days of food for every member of their family. Everyone desires the green numbers, as they signify those that will be served first. Pre-COVID-19, all three sets of numbers would be used. Now, the community is hesitant and even scared of leaving the house. Nobody can afford to be sick these days.

As a result, the numbers at the pantry are down. At least two sets of numbers and maybe three depending on the time of the month. Checks come out at the end and beginning of the month, and though there is always need, there is less need at those times. Those that do not understand the need may criticize those who rely on this place and call people that come here "entitled" or "lazy" as if poverty is only a myth or a matter of willpower. Better not to debate but instead continue to serve. There is always uncertainty in these neighborhoods.

When people arrive at this early hour of 6:00 am at this time of year, it is light outside and the birds are up and singing their songs. The neighborhood is quiet this time of day. The night shift people doing what they do went to bed recently, and those that needed to get to work are already gone. There is a stillness and, at another time of year (during the later fall and winter), it would be dark. See, poverty, like COVID-19, does not care what time of year it is and whether it is light or dark. Both do what they do, and, in this neighborhood, there is little pushback from those that live here. The residents and those that arrive are doing the best they can with what they have available.

Dennis is always present on the day this place is opening. A big man with dark eyes, he keeps watch over the numbers and the front entrance. He too comes for food for his family, but he also gives much to the organization as a volunteer. He greets people with a smile and maybe an elbow bump in this time of COVID-19. Those that gather here like appropriate hugs and touches, but in this time of the virus, it has decreased. The hugs are missed, and it is not known when they will return. Someone says,

"I'll give you twice the hugs when this is over," and they mean it. The people gather and Dennis gives out numbers in ones and twos—with a nod and a smile and, "You are welcome," to those who thank him. Small acts of kindness go a long way in a world filled with scarcity.

They continue to arrive a couple of hours before the place opens. They come in cars and trucks that have seen better days. Dents and scratches and sometimes loud exhausts spew blue smoke out the back end. Almost all have brown rust behind a wheel well or in front of the rear bumper that is bent from either being hit or bumping into something. Salt and water create a cancer on cars and trucks, slowly consuming the vehicles year by year— yet the vehicles bring people. Some are single families, and some are double or tripling up. Having a vehicle is a luxury when you must haul six bags of groceries for your family. If there is no automobile, people walk or even ride a bike. Just getting by . . .

They gather from all over the city. This place is not required to serve one zip code and so they come—many with Black and Brown skin. Many languages are spoken here—at last count, eleven, including sign language. See, hunger does not care what language you speak, and the only solution to hunger is food and nourishment. Language never stopped this place from providing what they can with what they have. Somehow, it all works out. The people are fed, and there is enough and seemingly abundance if there is sharing. The families are small, and the families are large. Some families are directly related while others are related through kinship or culture. The sharing not only pertains to food but to place. Some have multiple families living under one roof. People are doing what they have to do to get by and to survive.

One gathering place in one city, not as an anomaly, but as an everyday occurrence. See, poverty is all around this city, and in cities across this country, where there is a stark mark for those that have and those that have not. Better not be on the latter side—but the line between the two groups is shrinking. There are more people out of work and more people in need. Those that live in this way know how it goes, but what about the newcomers to poverty? Will they know how it goes and where to go and how to make the connections to survive? Time will only tell, and it is in the uncertainty of this virus that we must come together, to share resources and to hope.

This is our community, and we gather.

The Patient Told Me, "You Cannot Take Care of Me. You're Black, and I Don't Like Black People." How Do You Respond?

Victor Redmon, MD

Dr. Redmon, an MCW resident in Medicine and Pediatrics, serves on the diversity and inclusion committee for residents. In this essay, he shared two experiences where he struggled to know how best to deal with racism he encountered in the hospital.

The year of 2020 has been one for the ages. I have been more cognizant of reading articles addressing intolerance, injustice, and microaggressions this year, more so than in years past. A medical student on our service recently asked me particularly good questions about accountability and when to speak up, either for yourself or others, when your colleagues or patients make insensitive remarks. I do not know if I gave him the best answer at the time, partly because I do not know if there is one right answer.

A patient care story:
A woman with infections and confusion

In medical school, I was taking care of a woman during my third-year internal medicine clerkship. She was Caucasian and in her sixties. She was admitted overnight with confusion, and we found she had pneumonia, a urinary tract infection, and encephalopathy.

The next morning, I walked into the room alone and introduced myself along with my role on the team. She took one look at me and said, "You cannot take care of me. You're Black, and I don't like Black people." I paused, and then she rambled on about other things that didn't make much sense. I asked permission to examine her, and she stopped talking and let me perform my examination.

Once I was done, I thanked her and told her I would see her later in the day. She said, "Okay, but I don't like Black people."

We treated her infections, and her confusion cleared. She became more coherent and "with it." The next day when I went to see her, she greeted me with a, "Good morning."

I replied back, "Good morning. It looks like you are feeling better today."

She said, "Yes, I am. Who are you?"

I realized that she did not remember our first encounter, so I reintroduced myself. She thanked me and the team for our treatments. The rest of the encounter with her was very pleasant, and we discharged her home eventually.

I keep thinking about how and why I handled this encounter the way I did. I knew the patient was delirious from her active infections and hospitalization. Does that give her a pass for what she said to me? How much truth was in her words? I never told anyone on my team about what she said to me. Not my fellow third-year student colleague, not my intern, not my senior resident and not my attending. Why did I choose not to?

Another story:
A difficult homeless veteran and an intern's response

During my second year of residency, I was the senior resident of one of the medical ward teams at the VA. We had a patient who was notorious for his abuse of the health system, bigotry, and sexism. He was homeless, and every time he was admitted to the hospital, it was a saga to get him discharged. If you worked at the VA long enough, you knew this guy by name alone. You were either on his good side or his bad side. I had taken care of him several times in the past, starting when I was still a medical student. The patient and I had a good doctor-patient relationship, and he was never disrespectful to me. I wish I could say that for the ways he treated others.

My third day on the team, my intern following this particular patient came back to the room laughing. I chuckled and asked him what was so funny. "Oh Mr. So-and-So being Mr. So-and-So," he replied, "he's not so bad if you're on his good side." The patient had been medically ready for discharge for weeks, and we had been working with social work and case management to find him a place to stay since he required home oxygen therapy.

After rounds, our attending went to speak with the patient alone to basically tell him that he would be discharged the following day, and he could not stay in the hospital any longer. My intern was very nervous about how this would affect his own relationship with the patient. I told him that the patient would be more likely to be mad at the attending, but I offered to be there for him if he needed me. My intern declined and said, "I'll just see how it goes."

The next day, my intern came in laughing again. "Mr. So-and-So is still Mr. So-and-So." I took it as a positive sign and moved on. During rounds, our attending asked how Mr. So-and-So was doing today. My intern said, "He's fine, nothing has changed medically. But he hates you," referring to my attending. My intern then said, "He says he never wants to see 'that Brown, Jihad ***********
again.'"

This statement was wrong on so many levels. My intern laughed it off. Our attending, of Indian descent, was silent for a moment, but then said, "Well unfortunately, he doesn't have a choice." I looked around, and the rest of the team (the other intern and two medical students) was dead silent.

Internally, I was an emotional wreck. I felt anger, remorse, shock, and regret all at once. I didn't know how to respond at that moment. I was with people I had not grown comfortable with yet, so I froze and didn't respond at all.

As a team, we moved on and finished rounds. The patient was discharged later in the day without much drama. The following day was switch day for both the interns and the attending, so I had a whole new team.

I kept wondering what would have been the right thing to do. Approaching the patient about what he said would have not been a battle worth fighting. However, I never approached anyone else on the team, either, about what was said, how they felt, and how we could have done things differently. I missed an opportunity to point out intolerance and injustice and to take a stance on a perpetuated culture that needs to end. I feel like I failed my team. I feel like I failed as a leader.

There is no one "right way" to deal with these issues, but we must address them

I could continue to write about countless stories that are similar and worse than that which I discussed above. Whatever personal accounts or stories that my friends and colleagues have experienced, these types of encounters happen every single day. Often, we are silent and decide not to say anything so we can keep the peace. I no longer regret being timid in those moments. I felt I was doing what was necessary to "survive" and progress to where I want to be in life. I imagine that others have taken similar stances for similar reasons.

I do not think there is one "right or wrong" way to handle these situations, but I do think it is a reflection on how little improvement we have made as a society in addressing these issues.

I realize now that it is not about me or one person at a given time. It's about all of us as a society. As a medical society, we have a significant impact on our communities, especially the marginalized communities. It does not matter if you are a medical student, a physician, a nurse practitioner, a physician assistant, a nurse, a medical assistant, a physical therapist, or a speech therapist. You have a voice. You have a platform to use to speak out against injustice, intolerance, and microaggressions that we too often meet in our work environment.

I am far from perfect, and I do not pretend to be free of my own implicit biases. I hope to further an inclusive culture. I want to be called out if I am being insensitive or have a moment of intolerance, because that's how we grow as humans. I hope that I can learn from my failures and successes. At the same time, I hope others can learn from my experiences and their own experiences as well.

A challenge to all of us

We can no longer stay silent about these issues. There is a lot of work to be done, but small, simple steps eventually lead to larger ones. I intend to start speaking up for my colleagues; especially for my trainees and students, who are in a particularly vulnerable period in their life. I hope we are not alone.

Milwaukee is Special; Let's Make Some "Good Trouble, Necessary Trouble"

Adina Kalet, MD MPH

Shortly after Congressman John Lewis died of cancer, Dr. Kalet wrote this essay focusing on the importance of medical educators and health policy advocates to make "good trouble" by focusing on the needs of the disadvantaged communities in our midst.

On the day of his funeral, John Lewis, the civil rights warrior and seventeen-term congressman from Georgia's 5th Congressional District, published a love letter to the American people in the *New York Times*. He wrote his inspired and inspiring essay while dying of cancer, knowing that the country he loved was in crisis. *"You filled me with hope about the next chapter of the great American story when you used your power to make a difference in our society."*

Lewis reminds us that "Redeeming the Soul of Our Nation" will require a "long view" which, I believe, is also our approach as we redesign medical education to create a new physician workforce. Doing meaningful and important work is a process, not an outcome. As an ancient Jewish ethicist reminds us, we are not responsible for finishing the work of "perfecting the world," but neither are we free to stop trying.

Our home: Milwaukee is a very segregated city

We have some complex work to do in our own hometown.

Milwaukee has the long-standing, dubious distinction of being among the worst places in America to be Black. A Black child born into poverty in Milwaukee is more likely to continue to be poor than in any other large city in the country. Deeply entrenched, persistent and concentrated poverty, extreme racial segregation, and exclusionary zoning or "redlining" have been blamed for the poor social mobility for our Black children. There are endless, complex explanations for this "special" status.

Research studies confirm that health disparities are both directly and indirectly linked to these social determinants of poor health. Scientists from multiple institutions have identified that the incremental, accumulated physical effects of racism over a lifetime contribute to health inequities. Recently, this disparity has included the disproportionate illness and death of Black Milwaukeeans from COVID-19. No matter how you assess the current situation, things appear bleak.

Yet, John Lewis—a Black man who lost as many battles for racial justice as he won and who was beaten and arrested over fifty times for engaging in militantly nonviolent protest against racial injustice—was optimistic when he died.

Lewis believed in us. He exhorted us to be aspirational. He wrote, *"Ordinary people with extraordinary vision can redeem the soul of America by getting in what I call good trouble, necessary trouble."* It is time for those of us in medical education to do some significant envisioning. But where do you look for leadership? Inward?

Time to make some good and necessary trouble

As the Director of the Robert D. and Patricia E. Kern Institute for the Transformation of Medical Education, I am always on the lookout for opportunities to think boldly and make a bit of good and necessary trouble!

I am proud of MCW and its 125-year history of being an anchor institution in Milwaukee and the region. MCW's president, John Raymond, reviewed a list of the substantive ways in which MCW has been an exemplary institutional citizen of the city, the region, and the state over the past decade. He also invited all of us to join in the conversation and contribute to the MCW 2025 Strategic Framework, as we set a new vision and as we rise to current challenges; we must *". . . think boldly and to share how you would reimagine MCW."* How do we prepare to make changes?

Be bold, set audacious goals

Many years ago, my mentor diverted me from an unproductive tirade by saying, playfully, *"Don't get mad. Get data."* This admonition literally was the birth of my academic career. Below, I offer an example of people who will change Milwaukee by first gathering data.

The African American Leadership Alliance MKE (AALAM) was founded in 2017 to link influential individuals dedicated to making Milwaukee a place where African Americans thrive. AALAM has set the audacious goal of putting Milwaukee into the top ten US cities for African Americans by 2025! That is when our current first-year students will be interns.

Recognizing the need for benchmarks for their work and seeking to identify the levers to drive positive change, AALAM commissioned the UW-Milwaukee Center for Economic Development (UWMCED) to produce the study, "The State of Black Milwaukee in National Perspective: Racial Inequality in the Nation's 50 Largest Metropolitan Areas." The study was funded by the Greater Milwaukee Foundation.

As part of their work, the UWMCED team created a "Composite Index of African American Well-Being." The index synthesized thirty indicators of community well-being, typically studied individually—for example, employment, income, poverty, social and community health, and conditions specific to youth and children—into a single number allowing big picture comparisons and holistic analyses across large metropolitan areas of the country. *Milwaukee ranked fiftieth out of fifty.*

The study pinpoints three interrelated drivers for change:

- Reducing racial segregation
- Enhancing Black educational attainment
- Increasing the numbers of Black executives and managers at Milwaukee companies, including MCW

These actions will help make strides toward racial equity. For AALAM and the rest of us, it is a call to action, a time to make some good and necessary trouble.

Building trust and taking action

On July 22, 2020, Doctors Lenard E. Egede and Rebecca J. Walker from the MCW Division of General Internal Medicine Center for Population Health published a perspective in the *New England Journal of Medicine* identifying six recommended action items for mitigating structural racism. Directly in our Kern Institute lane is the recommendation to *"be consistent in efforts by health systems to build trust in vulnerable communities."*

How do we build trust? We must commit to long-term, trustworthy partnerships in "pipeline to the health professions" programs that will measurably accelerate the diversification of the health workforce in Milwaukee. We must intentionally and assertively recruit and support students, residents, faculty, and staff from underrepresented minority (URM) communities, making special effort to identify those from economically deprived backgrounds. And as our leaders are seeking to do, we must support, listen to, and engage with all of MCW's URM community—including all levels of staff—to be the kind of employer where everyone feels they belong, have an influence, and can create a meaningful work life. This will require carefully examining how we traditionally have approached fairness, as compared with equity, in admissions and hiring processes.

How do we prepare our trainees to practice medicine so that it is experienced by communities as trustworthy? Beyond a curriculum which provides the critical historical context for the distrust of the healthcare system by vulnerable communities, we must provide meaningful ways for our students and residents to work with and in communities. I have been involved with many "patient-as-teacher" programs. These programs train and employ community members to be medical school teachers. With their active participation, for instance as standardized patients, students can learn clinical material, practice skills, and receive critical feedback. With community guides and coaches, students and residents can contribute to research and engage in community social action. These experiences need to be substantive, rigorous, and longitudinal, allowing for the development of strong, trustworthy relationships. This is making some good trouble!

In his essay, John Lewis wrote that he once heard the voice of Martin Luther King, Jr. on the radio. *"He said we are all complicit when we tolerate injustice. He said it is not enough to say it will get better by and by. He said each of us has a moral obligation to stand up, speak up and speak out. When you see something that is not right, you must say something. You must do something. . . . I urge you to answer the highest calling of your heart and stand up for what you truly believe."*

If we are truly committed to transforming medical education—as well as society at large—we must reshape our own community, focus on character and caring, and offer to partner with organizations, like AALAM, that carry visions of a better, diverse, equitable world. Our entire community will benefit.

Microaggression

Bruce H. Campbell, MD, FACS

Dr. Campbell, an otolaryngologist and narrative medicine advocate, wrote this essay about how one of his residents caught him in his own racism and taught him about microaggression.

I distribute a short story to the fifteen residents and students sitting around the conference table. They follow along as one of them reads aloud:

"One last blow, and, blind as Samson, the Black man undulates, rolling in a splayfooted circle. But he does not go down. The police are upon him then, pinning him, cuffing his wrists, kneeing him toward the van. Through the back window of the wagon—a netted panther."

I am working to integrate narrative into medical education. On this early morning, the ENT residents and a few medical students concentrate—heads down, brows furrowed—as they take turns reading aloud "Brute" by Richard Selzer, a riveting first-person short fictional story first published in 1982. An exhausted young surgeon must repair the gash on a prisoner's forehead in the middle of the night. Both the surgeon's frustration and his admiration of the patient escalate as the roaringly drunk Black man "spits and curses and rolls his head." After one last, unheeded demand to "Hold still!", the surgeon calmly sews the man's ears to the cart, wipes the blood from the man's eyes, and grins victoriously down into his face, a demeaning gesture the surgeon profoundly regrets many, many years later.

The reading ends and everyone's eyes widen. The trainees are well on their way to becoming surgeons, and I watched them squirm as they read the story from the surgeon's point of view. "So," I ask the group, "what are your reactions?" After a pause, the discussion flows. Residents nod knowingly, recalling difficult, late night encounters with uncooperative, ungrateful people. "God," says a resident close to completing her five-year training, "those situations are really frustrating. I know exactly how he feels." Some of the students—having never been in the ER with a drunk—wonder aloud, "But what do you actually do?" and "Do you think this is a real story? Did this really happen?" I break off the discussion at the end of the hour. Several thank me as they file out. We have all been given something to contemplate.

A couple of days later, one of the senior residents, Tristan, and I are in the operating room. "Dr. Campbell," he says, "Melissa was upset by the story."

"Really?" Although Melissa is a junior resident, she

should have already had similar encounters. "About the way the surgeon reacted?"

"Talk to her."

Later that day, I track her down. "Melissa," I ask, "do you want to talk?"

"Dr. Campbell." Her gaze is steady and she speaks very evenly. "I was really disturbed when the writer portrayed the Black man as an animal. It was awful."

Oh, my goodness. Melissa has a mixed-race heritage. She is a gifted writer and a gentle soul.

"Tell me more."

"I hated how the writer described the victim. I was upset. I called my parents to talk about it and they said I should talk to you. I wasn't going to. I didn't want to talk."

"Sorry," I reply. "Tristan ratted you out."

We spend time talking through the reading and her reaction. Where I had always viewed the story through the surgeon's eyes, she had immediately identified with the patient. "I apologize," I say. "I have always seen the victim's race as a placeholder."

"Not for me," she says.

As we talk, I think back. I have used "Brute" in teaching sessions before but cannot recall if other residents and students of color participated. If they did, were they upset, as well?

Without recognizing the harm, I have perpetuated a racist act of prejudice—a "microaggression"—a misstep that I commit more often than I realize. Melissa has reminded me that I am a late-career, white male surgeon who grew up in a certain time and place and bring my own preconceptions to every experience. Even as I continue to teach residents and students, I must remain open to what my trainees teach me, as well.

"I'll find a different story next time," I tell her. "Or maybe you can help me teach it in the future."

She smiles. "I'll think about that," she says as she checks her pager. "Excuse me. I've gotta go to the ER."

Dear White Colleagues

Ashley M. Hines

In the aftermath of the killings of Breonna Taylor, Ahmaud Arbery, and George Floyd, Ms. Hines wrote this open letter. At the time, she was the Diversity and Inclusion Manager in the MCW Office of Diversity and Inclusion.

"You took my spot!" a classmate said in response to hearing that I had been accepted into the freshman class at the University of Wisconsin-Madison. I sat stunned. I took her "spot." What does that mean? I didn't think there were any spots. At the time, I didn't understand the real meaning of these four words. Over a decade later, it now makes sense.

As a wife, mother, full-time work-from-home staff member during the COVID-19 pandemic, and a Black woman amid the unending pandemic of racism, I've avoided facing my deep pain, hurt, confusion, anger, and sadness because I must keep it all together. In this letter, I pause and candidly share my thoughts on our current time. I am not and will never speak for all Black people. I encourage you to read and to listen to the many stories of the Black experience.

Police brutality and other forms of systemic racism and structured inequity are being recognized and spoken about in ways I've never experienced, magnifying the brokenness of our country. A country built, with intention, on racism and a 401-year-old system of oppression. Unfortunately, the system is working as it was intended. Breonna Taylor, Ahmaud Arbery, and George Floyd are among the countless individuals who have lost their lives because this country was built by us and on us, not built for us. Their stories amplify the destructive nature of pervasive injustice. We aren't talking about statistics; these are lives.

Many of my white colleagues have asked what they can do to support me. Here are some of my thoughts. Again, I cannot speak for all Black people.

See me

Presenting evidence that racism exists is exhausting and painful. Please don't discredit my personal experiences. Also, the impact of slavery is still felt today and is not far removed from many Black families. I'd argue that slavery has evolved—exposed by the disproportionate number of Black and Brown people in our criminal system—but that's an entirely different conversation.

This is complex, uncomfortable work

If there were easy solutions to racism and the systemic racism it produces, the work would be done. Inside MCW, a focus on pursuing learning and increased awareness, interrogating our practices, policies, and procedures at all levels, and transforming our system with bold changes is essential. Outside of MCW, protesting, voting, and changes across all sectors must happen. You will be nervous; you won't always say the right thing, and you will make mistakes. Move forward in humility and don't allow guilt to stop you. Plug in where you can and keep going!

This is a marathon, not a sprint

I understand that a system that has thrived for centuries will not change overnight. As the saying goes, "slow down to go faster."

It's not enough to not be a racist

We must be anti-racist. A Black woman recently posed a question to white folks, "What are you doing to make sure your children don't kill mine?" This is not the time to play it safe. Please don't be silent. People's lives depend on your commitment, voice, and thoughtful use of your unearned privileges.

Be in it with us

Acknowledge we are grieving, processing, and healing. Hold space for us to share and be patient and understanding if we can't do this every day.

Racism isn't new to me. In fact, like many people who identify as African-American and Black in the United States, it's an inescapable reality. I recognize some people haven't had to think about racism at all and do not know the fear (or have not experienced the fear) elicited by its deadly impact. The, "You took my spot!" comment hurt me for a long time. I carried it with me and struggled with impostor syndrome and non-belongingness. For me, implicit in her comment was a belief that she deserved something she had not earned simply *because* she was white. The sting of her comment drove me to work harder to prove my value to white people, to prove I deserved to be there and to prove I deserve to be here. But such continued comments and the deaths of unarmed Black people tell me that I can never prove myself sufficiently to overcome the biases and inequities built into a racist social system. Black Lives Matter is about Black people owning our inherent worth in a system that tells us differently.

I'm writing this letter on June 19, 2020. Today, we celebrate Juneteenth and recognize the last group of African Americans freed after the Civil War. This is Independence Day for African Americans and Blacks. Yet, we aren't free from the disparaging and multigenerational impacts of racism and slavery. Still, we celebrate because we are a resilient and empowered people.

So yes, I am hurt, confused, angry, and sad. And yet, most days, hopeful. I am grateful to work at MCW and heartened by our commitment to be an anti-racist organization. The work needed to undo the legacy of racism is difficult, and I believe it will get done. It must get done.

An Open Letter to My Colleagues

Loren Nunley, MD MBA

In the aftermath of the killings of Breonna Taylor, Ahmaud Arbery, and George Floyd, Dr. Nunley wrote this open letter to his colleagues about an experience he had as a teenager. He gave permission to have his letter reprinted in the Transformational Times. At the time, he was a fellow in Infectious Diseases at MCW.

I am a Black man.

Ten days after my sixteenth birthday, I caused a car accident (with minimal damage and no injuries). As I made a sharp turn in the pouring rain, I lost control, hitting another vehicle stopped at a red light. Witnesses included two police officers. I was immediately ordered to step out of my vehicle. My white friend in the passenger seat was ordered to get out and stand across the street. Upon silently complying with the order, I was slammed against my own car. Moments later, still silent, I found my face, bloodied, on a curb with something heavy on the back of my neck. It was the knee of the police officer trapping my head against the curb as I struggled to breathe. I am fortunate. It wasn't for nine minutes. I was not murdered. But I will never forget the weight of that knee on my neck.

George Floyd isn't a stranger. You work with him. You know him.

I am George Floyd.

This does affect you. So how will you affect it?

There are many meaningful actions you can take and places you can contribute. Consider these opportunities as starting points, but you can take it upon yourself to do further research on how you can help work towards positive change.

- Research organizations that are making a difference in communities of color. Donate, volunteer, and get to know the people involved.
- Support legal services and social service agencies that focus on communities of color.
- Educate yourself by reading articles and books on the Black experience.
- Support your friends, neighbors, and colleagues.

From the bottom of my heart, thank you for your kind consideration.

Be courageous,
Loren

Perpetuum Mobile

Keng Moua

This is an original poem by MCW-Milwaukee medical student Keng Moua. The music term, "perpetuum mobile," refers to "extended passages that are meant to be played in a repetitious fashion, often an indefinite number of times."

She told me
"You speak English really good"
I didn't have the heart to tell her
That I had lost my native tongue
Or that I only knew English

So I did what I always do
And laughed

He told me
"You're Japanese, you must love sushi"

I didn't have the heart to tell him
That I wasn't Japanese
Or that I hate sushi

So I did what I always do
And laughed

They told me
"Go back to your country"
I didn't have the heart to tell them
That I was born in the hospital down the street
Or that I grew up in this neighborhood

So I did what I always do
And laughed

Ahmad Arbury, George Floyd, Rayshard Brooks,
Jacob Blake, Breonna Taylor, Elijah McClain and
countless others
    I don't have the heart
    To think of how many more
    Or when it will end

So I did what I never do
And cried

Community Reflections: What's one concept you understand more deeply now?

Jessica Sachs, an MCW-Milwaukee medical student, submitted this response:

Recently, I have gained a better understanding of white apathy. White apathy is only knowing the names of Black men and women who lose their lives to police violence if they receive sufficient media attention. White apathy is the ability to choose when we want to engage with racial injustice and when we want to look away. White apathy is asking our Black peers to teach us about racism instead of doing the work ourselves, and failing to recognize the privilege of studying rather than experiencing it directly.

We must unlearn our legacy of silence and commit to continuously fight for racial justice.

Community Reflections: When you think back on Summer 2020, what will you remember?

Debra Nevels, the Community Engagement Program Manager for the MCW Cancer Center, submitted this response:

Coming to the reality that some, not all, people fear me simply because of the color of my skin. Realizing that there are so many more that do not see me in this light. Identifying so many that may not be family or friends but are allies in this fight. Committed to making sure that racism is not permanent.

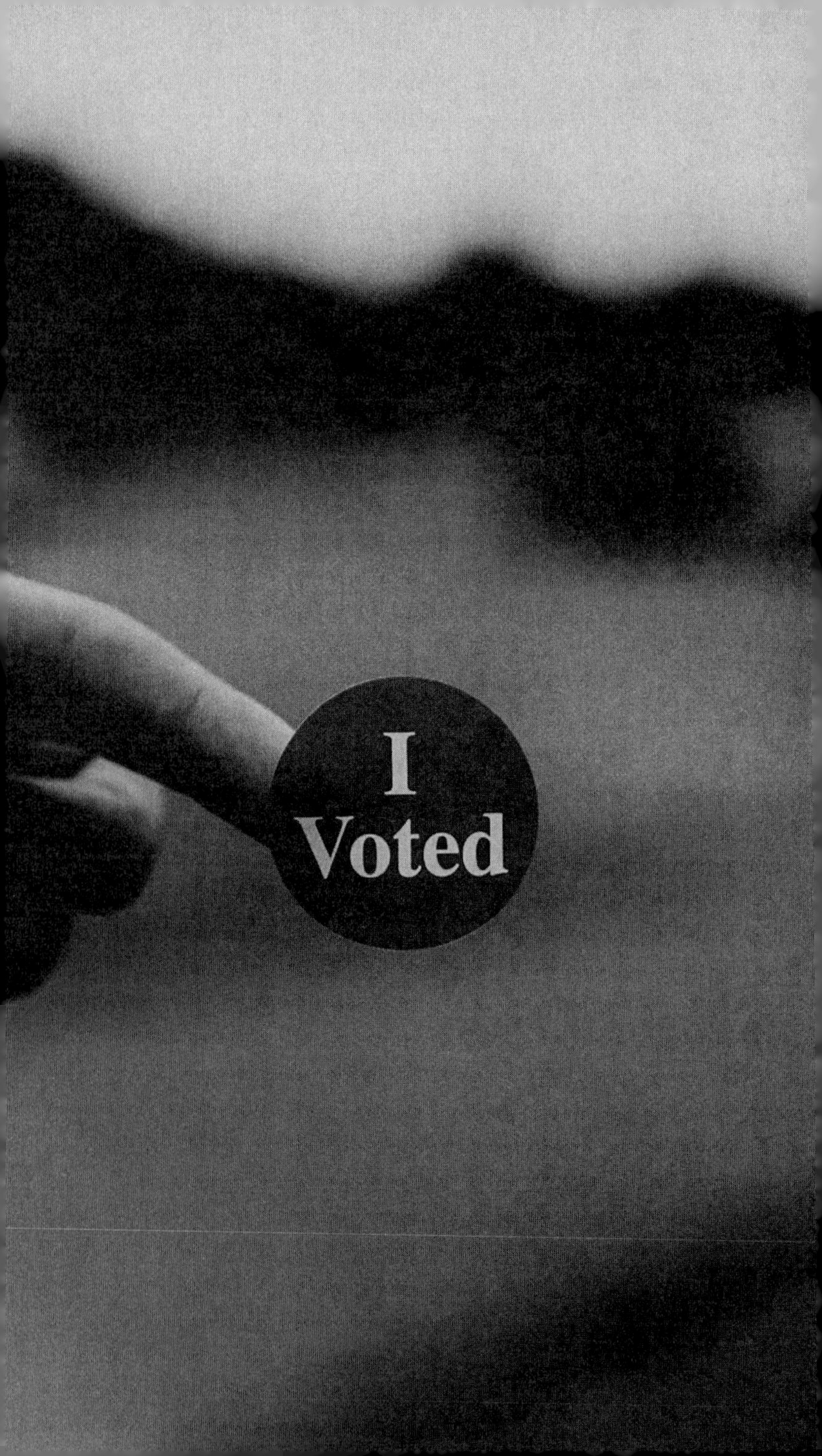
I
Voted

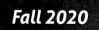
Fall 2020

The Lonely Only: Physician Reflections on Race, Bias, and Residency Program Leadership

Camille B. Garrison, MD

Dr. Garrison wrote this essay about implicit bias and microaggressions that she had experienced. This essay, which also appeared in the journal, Family Medicine, *won the 2020 MCW President's Prize for Medical Creative Writing.*

My earliest memory of wanting to become a doctor was when I was eight years old. Dr. R. saw me watching him intently as he examined my little brother's ear. He peeked up at me over the otoscope and asked if I wanted to look. From that day forward, he inquired at subsequent visits if I still wanted to be a doctor, which led to more detailed discussions about what I would need to do to achieve my goal. Dr. R. probably didn't know how important those discussions were for me, but I sensed that he believed that I too could become a physician one day. Throughout my childhood, I worried that it would be difficult for a person who looked like me to become a physician, as I didn't personally know any physicians with my racial identity.

As a child, my image of a physician was an Indian man, like Dr. R. I identify myself as an African-American female physician, and I am often in situations where I am the only person bearing that identity in the room. I consider myself the "Lonely Only" because I am the only African-American faculty in my residency program, the only one among our family medicine residency program leadership, the only one on our hospital leadership team, and the only one in most instances when it comes to my role as physician. I've had numerous experiences with implicit and explicit bias and personal racism in the workplace and have experienced the emotional burden that comes with being the Lonely Only. My responses to these experiences have evolved as I have progressed in my career, through gaining a better understanding of the environments in which I've worked, and in finding my voice to affect that environment when racial issues emerged. Now nine years post-residency, I am the program director for an urban underserved family medicine residency program in one of the most segregated metropolitan cities in the United States. My experiences as a Lonely Only have led me to accept responsibility for addressing issues of racism and the associated health disparities we see in medicine in my role as program director, specifically through resident education, faculty development, patient care, and community engagement. I strive to address these issues daily.

A few years ago, I had an encounter with one of my colleagues that served as the catalyst for me in confronting issues of bias and racism within my own program. I was having small talk with another faculty in our precepting room and mentioned something I recently saw on the news. There was a shooting at a private suburban school, and I mentioned how shocking this was to me. My colleague wasn't shocked at all. As I sat there wondering why he wasn't surprised, he answered my question. "Well, more and more Black kids go to that school now." My immediate response was, "Well, they never said anything about the race of the shooter." He looked at me with a blank stare as if there was nothing wrong with his comment. I was mortified, embarrassed, and furious all at the same time. I was concerned for the resident sitting next to me and wondered if any medical students or staff could've been passing by hearing our discourse. I was also saddened by thinking about the patients that he took care of and if he really held the belief that more Black people equates to more violence.

The rest of the evening, I reflected on several experiences I had in the past as a physician where I was reminded of my race. I remembered my former faculty taking a piece of cellophane tape and sticking it on my skin to see if any pigment came off on the tape. I thought about the times that I'd been referred to as "home-girl" in professional settings by other faculty members. I thought about the time when one of my advisees told me that she felt intimidated by my feedback because she didn't have much previous experience with Black women and "how we are," demonstrating what she meant by smacking her lips and giving me a quick neck roll. These memories brought forth so many unresolved emotions and feelings of sadness, anger, and shame (for being silent), that I knew this time I had to do something.

The following week, I called the program director to inform him of my concern and asked that he be present for the meeting with my colleague. Our meeting started with an explanation of how the comments made me feel as an African-American woman and mother of African-American boys. I talked about our predominantly African-American patients and staff and how they might have perceived his comments. He repeatedly stated that he didn't mean to offend me and that he didn't see me in "that way." I explained to him the way I see myself and the way I believe the world sees me, as an African-American woman first. I talked about how differently people might think of him when he walks outside of our clinic doors, as they might assume he's a doctor, while I might not be considered a physician at all, simply because of my race. It was at that moment that he started to understand, and he apologized.

Did my colleague intend to offend me by his comment? I don't think so. But that's how implicit bias works. If we are not in tune with our personal biases and how to stop biased thinking as it occurs, those thoughts will eventually be expressed in the open. I felt empowered after speaking to my colleague that day, and it helped prepare me for future encounters, as I began to see incidents where I was reminded of my skin color as opportunities to intervene, rather than as burdens.

Early in my career, I experienced the friction that can come rom leading these discussions and acknowledged that at times it comes with personal costs. In the past, I felt isolated when colleagues tried to discourage me from having discussions at our program about racism and felt misunderstood when sharing my personal experiences with racism. I even felt overlooked when leadership opportunities became available and wondered if that had to do with my race. I started thinking, "Why do I always have to be the one initiating conversations about racism and biases?" until I shifted my focus to what was most important for our patients. Our patients need providers who understand the racial factors affecting their health and who can address them in an equitable way, limiting bias. As program director, I've found ways to teach our physician team that learning about the impact of racism is imperative to addressing the health disparities that our patients face. I teach that these disparities can be addressed through individual patient encounters, mentoring underrepresented minority residents, implementing curricular changes in our community medicine education, enhancing community engagement activities, and leading related resident didactics and faculty development sessions.

It took some time before any formal teaching occurred in my program after my implicit bias incident. I was a more junior faculty member when the event took place. However, one year later, I became the program director and started making small changes within our program, teaching more on our underserved patient population and health disparities. I later hosted discussions regarding the physician role and the Black Lives Matter movement, facilitated a clinic-wide viewing of the *Milwaukee 53206* documentary (set in my childhood neighborhood) highlighting inequities in incarceration rates, and poverty, and allowed for a new resident-led social justice group. In 2017, I partnered with another physician working in a similar residency program setting (who is also an underrepresented minority) and we developed a workshop on racism that we facilitated at both of our programs this past year.

It has been heartening to see the influence of efforts in these areas, as our residents and faculty have taken steps to learn, discuss, teach, and practice medicine with better understanding of racism and bias. In some ways, I have come to accept being the Lonely Only, now willing to share my experiences as an African-American physician, because for our program, racism has become a topic that is open for discussion and intervention. I have learned how to navigate being a Lonely Only through seeking opportunities to build skills to recognize unresolved emotions and by using coaching, mentoring, and other resources when confronting racism, both indirectly and directly. I have chosen to fully embrace the responsibilities of being the Lonely Only, as the downstream impacts of my efforts can have enormous implications for the care of my patients and the health of my clinic community.

May I Drink Coffee?

Olivia Davies

Dr. Davies, who was a senior medical student at the time when she created this essay, reflected on how the pandemic was disrupting the process of interviewing for residency.

I've tried three different Zoom setups, four if you count the one from my couch that I joke about. One of my friends has a bouquet of flowers set stage left on her screen, just in sight. I play with the tilt of my monitor to see if I can show the top leaves of my split leaf philodendron which sits on the floor next to me. Staring at the white wall behind me through the screen monitor, I catch a glisten—is that grease? I turn around to examine it in real time, yup, grease. How did that even get there? To be fair, I am sitting next to the wall where our dinner table was just a mere two days ago, before I declared it my new interview spot.

"Do you have the *Milk Street Cookbook*?" my fiancé calls from the other room. I sigh, removing it from the stack underneath my laptop. I know I should be grateful he's making the grocery list this week (like he does almost every week), but doesn't he understand we only have so many laptop-sized books in this apartment to elevate the built-in camera? I realize using *Milk Street* as my laptop prop probably won't be sustainable.

One of my friends asked if I was planning to wear heels . . . I guess I hadn't thought of that. She smiles matter-of-factly and says, "I am, they make me feel put together, even if no one will see them." She has a point, I think. I stand up, shimmying out of the screen to go look for my suit jacket. Finally unearthing it from my closet, I gasp at how dated it looks. Were flashy gold buttons "in" five years ago? This won't play well on camera. I sit back down and start to look for a simple suit jacket online.

Reaching for my phone to text my friend back, I glimpse my half hunched over frame in the monitor. "I think I'll wear heels, too," I say, un-pretzel-ing my feet from beneath me and placing them firmly on the ground. Before setting down my phone, I fire off one more text, "Do you think it's okay to drink coffee?"

M1 Students React to COVID-19: Feeling Helpless, Seeking Knowledge, and Becoming Empowered

On May 15, 2020—while students were banned from attending in-person classes and ten days before George Floyd was killed in Minneapolis—medical students from all three MCW campuses joined together virtually to hear presentations on the current state of knowledge about SARS-CoV-2. Several students provided reactions to the session and stories of their lives at the time. Below is a selection.

Anna Janke—M1 MCW-Milwaukee

So many pieces of information I had previously taken as facts were flipped on their heads, as our panelists separated fact from fiction. . . . I had not realized that the transfer of information from virology/medical experts to popular press is a bit like the game "telephone" where facts and terms may get lost in translation. For example,

COVID-19 is a disease, rather than an infection; the infection is called SARS-CoV-2. Furthermore, some information spread by the media and laypeople on social media is downright false. Before this presentation, I had no idea that SARS-CoV-2 mutates more slowly than influenza due to the proofreading ability of its replicase complex … I was quite shocked to learn that "social distancing" and "six feet apart" will not, in fact, completely prevent the spread of SARS-CoV-2, as infected aerosols can stay in the air and travel for hours.

As my first year of medical school comes to an end, I am left with a lot more concerns than I started with, in all honesty. Partly from the pressures of medical school and partly due to holing up at home in the midst of an unprecedented pandemic, I struggle to find meaning in the monotony of my days. However, I do not have to look hard to find those for whom I care and those who care for me, whether it be my friends, fiancé, family, or faculty at MCW.

British Fields—M1 MCW-Milwaukee

I know a lot of people that have had COVID-19 and have thankfully recovered, but I also know many that have had to bury a loved one that died from COVID-19. [O]ne of my mentees' mom is a nurse that contracted the virus and ended up on a ventilator. Thankfully, she is recovering, but I say that to say healthcare workers are risking it all for us. However, the triumph in togetherness does come with a tragedy. I have seen many ignorant people banning together to break laws openly and they are handed a mask by authorities. However, when a Black man takes a jog, he's murdered, and his murderers were freely walking after the incident. . . . Or the countless videos of Black gatherings being physically forced to break up by officers. COVID-19 has brought on a sense of togetherness, but it's also allowed the nasty principles that this country was built on to flourish and has put more fear in my heart about people more than the bug causing this virus.

Megan Quamme—M1 MCW-Milwaukee

This virus has taken a huge toll on me in a very personal way. My roommate went on a trip in March 2020, right when all of the restrictions were just beginning. She just turned twenty-six and has not had any significant medical history. It was the first weekend of our spring break. [I was still out of town when] she returned. The next day she felt sick and was told to get tested by her workplace. The following day, March 15, 2020, we heard the news that she was positive for SARS-CoV-2.

At the time, I thought that she would be in quarantine for two weeks and then I would be able to go home. The following week, she went to the hospital for shortness of breath. A few days later, she had to call 911 on herself to be taken to the ER. Her saturation was 80% when she arrived at the ER. She was given oxygen and some asthma treatments and was sent home with an albuterol inhaler. She said she could barely walk ten feet down the hall to use the restroom for a few weeks. She went to her primary doctor three times for follow-up chest X-rays after her symptoms would not go away.

On April 20, 2020, she finally had her first fever-free day. On May 4, she officially tested negative for SARS-CoV-2.

What started as a week-long [spring break] trip turned into a seven-week quarantine. My roommate was alone. If her situation had gotten worse, she could have ended up on a ventilator or even died, alone in the hospital.

I dealt with a lot of guilt during that time, and still am. I wonder if I am the one who gave it to her and just didn't have any symptoms? I wonder if there was more I could do to support her? I wonder how I was so lucky to avoid getting infected, and being ill at the same time as her. I wonder how her health will be affected for the rest of her life. Her doctor told her she will likely always have exercise-induced asthma.

I feel that I have a responsibility to tell my story, but it often falls on deaf ears. The only people who want to hear it are those who listen. I find myself in a struggle between trying to be a leader of my community and to be outspoken about evidence and my story and protecting my own mental health and well-being.

Benjamin Hodapp—M1 MCW-Green Bay

The greatest personal challenge I have felt during this pandemic has been the lack of agency in being able to affect positive change for those at risk. I chose to enter medicine for this specific reason. As students, my colleagues and I are in the unique situation of being in a helping profession with little-to-no agency when it comes to serving the public in any tangible way. I have done my best to define ways I can assist those less fortunate, but it feels woefully inadequate. Now that we approach entering the clinic on June 1, 2020, I am concerned for the safety of my 'soon-to-be' patients. Will I be the one who possibly transmits the virus to them? The strain of the dichotomy to be involved in the healthcare response while protecting my patients (after all, I am only a student with little to offer) has been a challenge as we approach the clinic commencement.

The main takeaway from the three lecturers was simply: while we know a great deal about this virus and its components, we know very little about treatment, disease progression, and how it will proceed in the coming months. Caution is our number one friend in this time of crisis, and it was heartwarming to hear rational, incredibly well-educated people that I sincerely respect speak about how we should be approaching future steps with care.

Sarah Steffen—M1 MCW-Central Wisconsin

As a medical student, and therefore someone who has committed herself to the idea and importance of scientific evidence and evidence-based practices, and to keep people safe from harm, COVID-19 has brought to reality—perhaps at one of its most nightmarish levels— the idea that a significant portion of our society dismisses science, education, and the universal human need to have empathy and take care of one another.

I come from a small, rural, and definitely more conservative town in the state of Wisconsin, and my social media, in particular Facebook, has been flooded with conspiracy theories and misinformation from people who often post about "not wanting to blindly follow others, and wanting to think for themselves." But following scientifically proven information is not following blindly. How do you get others to realize there is a difference between scientific evidence and an opinion? How do you get them to care?

For me today, the biggest takeaways from this session quite simply revolved around the themes of scientific information and compassion. Scientific information that was from credible sources and experts of multiple fields, and the compassion that went side by side with presenting that information for how we can work towards a better future to take care of one another.

The Congruence in my Quest

Sherréa Jones, PhD

Dr. Jones, an MCW-Milwaukee medical student, created this essay describing her journey as a Black woman where few of her teachers looked like her. She shared her vision of a future where structural racism is no more.

What made you decide to actively pursue your career? Traditionally, when this question is posed to the majority of people, their response involves seeing someone congruent to themselves in the profession they are seeking. For many Black individuals in this country, our answer to this question is, overwhelmingly, because we do not.

I grew up in the inner city of Milwaukee, WI. I graduated from a severely underperforming school system, and I found myself, as a child, pregnant with my very own child. I was raised by a single Black woman in a family where I was surrounded by other single Black women, none of whom were in a career that aligned to the professional aspirations I was captivated by on Thursday night television. Sure, every child wants to be a superhero growing up, and eventually those dreams become more realistic. In contrast to some other children, these fictional characters served as my only visual source of hope for a career in medicine.

During my first semester at UW-Madison, I found myself engulfed in feeling ridiculous for wanting to be a physician. Here I was, at a nationally recognized research institution, with 40,000 other students of which only 2% were Black. Five years later, I matriculated as the only Black student within the entire Department of Biological Sciences at Marquette University. I remained the only Black student for the duration of my tenure as a PhD candidate. As you might imagine, my scholastic unpreparedness resulted in grave academic struggles. I felt intimidated, shamed, defeated, embarrassed, and increasingly believed myself inferior in intellect compared to my white peers.

When I was granted the opportunity to join the class of 2024 at the Medical College of Wisconsin, I decided I was going to own this experience. I made the conscious decision to be transparent about my personal and academic struggles, my feelings of ineptness and, most importantly, my intentionality about using my voice as a vehicle to speak for the disenfranchised. Moreover, I desired to utilize the uniqueness of my physical presence to be there for those seeking racial, socioeconomic, and/ or gender congruence in their aspirations. Being in the racially distinct faction, as a student, was no longer shocking to me, it was the anticipated norm. What I did find resounding was the glaring lack of visible support for Black students at one of the largest teaching hospitals in the state of Wisconsin. A campus with an ever-expanding and commanding presence directly adjacent to the city of Milwaukee, which is nationally referenced as one of the most segregated cities in the United States, and consistently leads the nation in having the largest race-based disparities in health, wealth, and incarceration rates.

During my first year of medical school, I was introduced to a parade of PhDs and MDs who were facilitating my education, yet only one of them (Dr. Erica Arrington) looked like me. Prior to starting school, I read about well-established mentorship programs in place at numerous institutions that are targeted to help Black students thrive. There was, however, nothing in place here at MCW.

Although I did not see a tangible support network for Black students at MCW—except for a small number of individuals (Dr. Jennifer McIntosh, Jean Mallett, Dr. Cassie Ferguson, Dr. Michael Levas, Dr. Greer Jordan, Dr. Marty Muntz, and Dr. Malika Siker)—I refused to believe there was no interest in its erection. Similarly, I refused to believe that a hospital that cares for a largely impoverished and disadvantaged population, where many of its children were born, was a hospital that did not care to support the success of its future Black physicians in training. Furthermore, I refused to believe that an institution that welcomes over two hundred students each year (albeit only 4% are Black) did not have a proactive committee to offer resources and refuge to students who found themselves on academic probation, the frightening place I was in at the conclusion of my first semester at UW-Madison. I refused to believe that absolutely no one within administration, faculty, or staff had a genuine concern about the mental health and well-being of Black students.

Despite the daunting data and the countless conversations with my Black student colleagues surrounding feelings of isolation, frustration, and powerlessness, I am glad I held on to my skepticism. Through our activism and advocacy, we have been introduced to a village of physicians, administrators, staff, and non-Black students who have tremendous concerns about the deficiency of a culture that ensures the support and success of Black students. Through my student leadership roles, I have discovered a team of individuals that have launched a collective effort on shifting the paradigm at MCW built around anti-racist directives. There is a community at MCW that works tirelessly, while facing insurmountable organizational hurdles, against the structural inequalities that are systematically designed to perpetuate the failure of Black students that choose to enroll at MCW based on the advertised supportive nature of the program.

In discovering this assemblage, I have begun a personal quest to bring awareness to this community. Although this quest feels strikingly reminiscent of the imaginary characters I held on to in an effort to catapult me to a realistic place of actively pursuing my dreams, I unequivocally embrace the intangible ideal that, one day, the members of this community will be unapologetically and unashamedly empowered to speak up for Black students, visibly support Black students, and enforce palpable change for the betterment of the Black student experience at MCW.

It took over four hundred years to structure the system that anticipates my failure. I am well aware that I cannot unravel it in four.

The Truth About Trust

Adina Kalet, MD MPH

In the shadow of the first 2020 Presidential Debate between Donald Trump and Joseph Biden, Dr. Kalet wrote about how we measure and instill trust and trustworthiness in students and trainees.

"Anyone who doesn't take truth seriously in small matters cannot be trusted with large ones either."
—Albert Einstein

The first presidential debate this week has me thinking about the consequences of not being able to trust someone on whom you depend. We rely on our elected officials, like our physicians, to listen, have empathy, engage in respectful—even if sometimes heated—disagreements, make good judgements in very complex situations, have control over intense emotions and, most importantly, consistently tell the truth. To "trust someone" implies that we have confidence in that person, and believe that the individual will be capable, adaptable, and competent now and in the future—even when faced with novel, rapidly evolving circumstances, emotional and physical stressors, and unpredictable challenges.

While always in the background, trust ("entrustment" and "trustworthiness") has moved to the forefront in medical education. How we make these trust judgements in medical education—and in life—is worth a hard look.

How do we measure trustworthiness in trainees?

In their book, *The Question of Competence: Reconsidering Medical Education in the Twenty-First Century*, Hodges and Lingard point out that the discourse about what makes a "good" physician—a core responsibility of our work as medical educators—has moved through a series of distinct and overlapping eras over the past seventy years. In the Psychometric Era, we valorized measurable, highly standardized knowledge tests (e.g., MCAT, USMLE, and Board Exams). The next phase brought great enthusiasm for demonstrable, directly observable, and behaviorally measurable core clinical skills (e.g., oral exams, mini-CEXs, and OSCEs). Next, and to the frustration of many program directors, organizations introduced comprehensive, nuanced competency frameworks designed to capture and document each learner's developmental progress via new standards and milestones.

These changes reflect our evolving grasp of "quality" in medical education. As our understanding improves, we will uncover how to develop rich portfolios of assessment data for each of our trainees. But in the end, the data does not make high stakes decisions. We do. And these decisions require making trust judgements and having the courage to act on those judgements.

Trust judgement barriers and opportunities

Unfortunately, clinical faculty are not very good at assigning objective measures of competence. My colleagues and I spent years trying to get experienced clinicians to make reliable (reproducible) measurements of medical student clinical competence. Even with lots of fancy performance dimension, frame of reference, and behavioral observation training, experienced professionals are eccentric and resist standardization. This, I believe, is because there is no single "truth" about clinical competence.

Trust judgments are highly context-dependent and idiosyncratic. We tend to be internally consistent and we know a trustworthy resident when we see one. An experienced professional possesses a highly-honed identity and a strong sense of what a trainee must demonstrate to be trusted to care for "our" patients. Unfortunately, we disagree with our colleagues on when individual trainees can be entrusted to "fly solo" and independently care for patients. Gingerich has challenged us to embrace this disagreement and see it as a strength rather than a weakness.

Furthermore, experts are also context-dependent! As we collect and collate more and more data from larger, diverse pools of experts, we must ensure that trust judgements are appropriately interpreted to protect students from the vagaries of any individual's bias. This is what van der Vleuten and others call a Program of Assessment for Learning. Ultimately, trained competence "judges" will be charged with making final high stakes assessments regarding decisions such as advancement and graduation. These judges will determine if, based on solid evidence, we can trust a learner to consistently "do the right thing, at the right time, for the right person, and for the right reason" in their next phase of training.

Moving from theory to action

Social and cognitive psychology researchers suggest that competency judges need to both understand the value and limits of the objective data (e.g., exam scores don't predict clinical skills competence, but they do predict future exam scores) and should explore and develop their judgement "sense." This sense of who to trust is highly dependent on an individual's characteristics, experiences, and biases. Knowing thyself, in particular understanding one's biases, is crucial because if we are cognizant of them and have integrity, we can make adjustments, "forcing" ourselves to slow down our thinking, toggle to a more analytical rather than intuitive deliberative strategy, when we are in danger of making an error. This takes work, discipline, and practice with feedback.

There is much interesting work to be done to ensure we have trustworthy physicians. Fundamentally, most of us make our trust judgments based not on what students know or can do (we can always teach that stuff), but on who they are as people. Do they always tell the truth even when it leaves them in a "bad light?" Do they admit when they missed a physical exam finding or forgot to check a lab or failed to follow up on something? Do they take the time to listen, attend to details, interact with empathy and kindness, even when stressed emotionally? Do they strive to improve rather than rest on their laurels or test scores? Do they seek to understand the perspectives of others? How do they handle being wrong or making a mistake? Can they sincerely apologize?

We are accountable to society to make defensible promotion and graduation decisions based on each learner's competence and trustworthiness. These shifting concepts are difficult to measure. We pledge to engage in the ongoing discourses and learn how best to make difficult, discerning judgements.

A "Sermon" for Medical Students About Civic Character

Mark D. Schwartz, MD

In this invited essay, Dr. Schwartz, who leads pre- and post-doctoral fellowship programs in population health and health policy at New York University, shared a series of lessons he has learned and offered a three-pronged challenge to today's medical students.

"If individual character is what we do when no one is looking, civic character is what we do when everyone is looking!"
—Eric Liu "Citizen University"

I remember the excitement and fear of drinking from the fire hose as a medical student in the 1980s. I was aware of, but could not fully understand, how the

AIDS epidemic was shaping and honing my professional identity, just as the current pandemic is shaping yours.

In this moment when the country is sick and suffering—when our health, our economy, and democracy are threatened and when science itself is being undermined—we need to impact the world beyond our next exam, our next rotation, our next patient, or our next scientific hypothesis.

Given the situation we are in, let's talk about what it means to be civically engaged physicians and scientists in this new world. Here are some simple but profound questions I have been living in, wrestling with, and trying to answer:

- Given our positions, capabilities, and resources, what are our responsibilities? And for whom are we responsible?
- What are our roles as civic physicians, civic scientists, and civic healers?
- How can we use our professional roles and power to strengthen democracy?

I can't tell you what your answer should be, but I do know that we need to think bigger.

Physicians have privilege and tremendous, untapped power. Power is misunderstood and mistrusted, yet there is no greater mechanism for positive change than through the harnessing of power and creating civic action. Power calls physicians to be positive agents of change in our communities.

Where and how do we begin?

I can guess what you are thinking. Listen, I get it. I am a doctor, a professor, a researcher, and a leader. I would put my "To-Do" list up against anyone's! I know how unthinkable it is to add one more task. It is overwhelming enough to develop into the best doctor or scientist you can be.

Besides being incredibly busy, I hear other reasons why physicians and scientists are hesitant to engage in strengthening our democracy. Here are three of them:

- Who can fight big money?
- Science and politics don't mix!
- It's not my job.

Let me unpack these with you.

Myth #1: We shouldn't engage in strengthening democracy because, "Who can fight big money?"

Undoubtedly, our democracy is driven by money and power. How can the rest of us ever have a voice? How can we not throw up our hands in cynicism and despair when we see how big oil, big banks, and big medicine turn policies, laws, and regulations in their favor? Here are two reasons why I am optimistic about your chance to make changes.

The first is that you have more power than you think. As voters, we exercise a vital act of civic power, and forming, joining, and aligning forces supercharges your civic power. Organizations like the American Medical

Association, American Hospital Association, or the Association of American Medical Colleges are out there every day, shaping how we educate, train, and practice medicine and science. When you align with your school's advocacy agenda, national student organizations, and professional societies, your voice is amplified. Take advantage. As Samuel Adams, who incited the Boston Tea Party, famously said: "It does not take a majority to prevail... but rather an irate, tireless minority, keen on setting brushfires of freedom in the minds of men."

The second reason why I am optimistic about your chances is that culture eats policy for lunch every day. Although policy includes the levers of public laws and regulations, culture—our norms, civic ideals, beliefs, habits, and practices—shapes our society's norms, values, and the spirit of democracy. Culture is tied to our "civic character." "If individual character is what we do when no one is looking, civic character is what we do when everyone is looking!" Civic character and behavior are contagious. If you doubt this, look around the country and notice how different regions of the US have responded differently to the pandemic and our emerging social conversations.

We mimic what we see—what we do grows and becomes social norms. We are not stuck in traffic—we are traffic. We are part of the ecosystem we create. Democracy is not a machine, but a garden that needs active tending; like a garden, it needs water, sunlight, planning, understanding and respect of cycles, weeding, and adaptation.

So, what can you do in your daily life to promote civic character and to close the gap between our ideals and our practice in this American democracy project? What does it mean to live like a citizen? John Wesley, the founder of Methodism in the 1700s, said:

> *"Do all the good you can,*
> *By all the means you can,*
> *In all the ways you can,*
> *In all the places you can,*
> *At all the times you can,*
> *To all the people you can,*
> *As long as ever you can."*

We need to think bigger!

Myth #2: We shouldn't engage in strengthening democracy because, "Science and politics don't mix!"

I teach a course on research methods each summer. Physicians and scientists venerate evidence. It is the ground on which we stand to do our work.

Were you as concerned as I was when it appeared that we were being pulled into an evidence-free world? Where truth becomes truthiness? Where each of us has our own dictionaries, our own encyclopedias, our own fragmented sources of evidence? Where national, scientific experts are pushed aside, data disappears, and evidence is ignored by our leaders?

I've got data, you've got data, we all have data. The power that you have, given your position, is to bring data to life with real, lived stories about how all this data plays out in the world and affects real people. With cameras on computers and phones, I have been inside the lives, families, and homes of many people suffering or worried about COVID-19. Yes, I have graphs of rising and falling cases and deaths, but I also have stories of loss, fear, hope, and how families and communities are coming together to help us heal, cope, and mourn. We are in a unique position to link data to stories. People will listen.

As citizen physicians and scientists, we have the responsibility to tell these stories, to bring the data and evidence to life. Each of us can strengthen our democracy by telling these stories to provide compelling, living context for our science, our data, and our evidence.

We need to think bigger!

Myth #3: We shouldn't engage in strengthening democracy because, "It's not my job to fix the country."

As a physician, my job is to help one person at a time when they come to see me.

Of course, only about 20% of health is affected by what doctors and scientists do in the office, the hospital, the lab. The other 80% is explained by our genes, our individual and civic behaviors, and the social determinants of health: where we grew up, learned, lived, worked, and played. These social determinants, with their history and the ways in which they are baked into society's institutions and structures, all drive the disparities that the twin pandemics of coronavirus and of racially-targeted violence and injustice have made undeniable.

Each day, we look into the eyes of the patient in front of us, to plumb the depths of a scientific problem, and stare into the computer to do the work we are preparing to do. That is difficult, valid, valiant, and vital work, but it is not enough. If we want to have a larger, more enduring impact, we must lift our eyes ~~from the patient, problem, and~~ computer and embrace the context and culture of our populations and communities.

We need to think bigger.

I teach a course on health policy, and so I get to watch students learn the language, the anatomy, and the physiology of how health policy is made. Their brows furrow and their faces get heavy as they grasp our crazy-complex policy machinery. They discern how policy is shaped by money and by self-interest.

But I have also seen their faces brighten after they pick a policy issue about which they are passionate, prepare and practice their advocacy pitch, and visit their representatives in Congress. They are surprised how easy and how important it is to engage as citizens and to leverage their power as future physicians and scientists. Participating in acts that engage our civic character strengthens our democracy and repairs the world, given our position, our capabilities, our resources, and our power.

A central tenet in Judaism is the responsibility we each have of *Tikkun Olam*, that is, to repair the world. We can't do the entire work, but we are called to do what is in our reach to knit together the broken ends and to partner in the work.

So, I leave you with the questions with which I began:

- Given our positions, capabilities, and resources, what are our responsibilities? And for whom are we responsible?
- What are our roles as civic physicians, civic scientists, and civic healers?
- How can we use our professional roles and power to strengthen democracy?

As a leading rabbinic scholar, Rabbi Tarfon, taught two thousand years ago, "It is not your responsibility to finish the work [of perfecting the world], but you are not free to desist from it either." My charge to you is to wrestle with these questions, connect with one another to engage the world where you can, and spend your careers searching for the answers. By developing and sharing your civic character, your work can lead to lasting change.

It's Tough Sledding Out There - Advocating for Safe Voting in Milwaukee

Christopher Davis, MD MPH

In the run-up to the 2020 elections, Dr. Davis emphasized the importance of voting and described the work of MCW's Safe Voting Task Force, a volunteer group that shared information and helped people register.

I co-chair MCW's Safe Voting Taskforce with Dr. Megan Schultz. Mostly a medical student- and resident-led endeavor, our efforts indeed generated some meaningful successes; however, our victories and defeats were, at the same time, both enlightening and infuriating. If we could have had our cake and eaten it too, we would have actively registered hospital and clinic patients, provided the entire community with safe voting information, and created a highly visible media messaging campaign. However, largely due to the politicization of voter registration, we couldn't bring home the gold. Nonetheless, I believe that we will still find ourselves on the medal stand, if only for dutifully fulfilling our civic responsibilities of promoting health and voting.

Our Successes

Those of us in healthcare must get our houses in order by casting ballots. To that end, we worked diligently with MCW's deans, center directors, chairs, and the Office of Graduate Medical Education to emphasize both the importance of voting and MCW's support for these efforts.

In an event hosted by the Kern Institute, Alister Martin (from the national VoteER Campaign), educated us and fielded questions about engaging hospital leadership to support patient voter registration. This effort led to direct patient engagement in both Children's Wisconsin's and Froedtert Hospital's Emergency Departments. Our student-led efforts even extended to Wausau, where MCW-Central Wisconsin medical student Hayden Swartz encouraged North Central Health Care and Ascension's local hospital systems to adapt the VoteER model to engage their patients to vote and vote safely.

Concurrently, our Safe Voting Task Force sought to engage a much broader audience. In order to avoid any appearance of "taking sides" in the process, MCW's Office of Government and Community Relations connected us with professionals at Badger Bay Management Company. In order to bypass partisanship, they suggested we reach out to the Wisconsin Public Health Association (WPHA) to take the lead for a statewide coalition of major health-related groups. WPHA's board quickly voted in favor of this and on October 8, 2020, we held the kickoff of "Vote Safe Wisconsin 2020." Keynoted by Dr. Susan Polan, the Associate Executive Director for Public Affairs and Advocacy of the American Public Health Association, the event helped secure pledges from numerous organizations in Wisconsin to support our efforts of ensuring that the public had the information it needed to vote safely. In addition to WPHA, the Wisconsin Medical Society, the Wisconsin Chapter of the American College of Emergency Physicians, and United Way of Wisconsin were engaged. By directly reaching at least 15,000 professionals across Wisconsin, MCW and WPHA has led a public health campaign to assure Wisconsin's citizens that they can vote and vote safely despite the surge in COVID-19 cases.

Lastly, MCW and the Kern Institute have continued to actively engage with our partners from MaskUpMKE, who launched MaskUp2Vote. This work combines the longstanding public health message of MaskUpMKE with information that voters might find useful in terms of where in Milwaukee to find free masks and the basics of voting safely during a pandemic. MaskUp2Vote also generated an animated public service announcement which features Bango (the mascot of the Milwaukee Bucks) and highlights the ongoing civic engagement and public support from the Milwaukee Bucks organization.

Our Failures

I am constantly reminded that the work of community engagement and uplifting our patients can be a slow and arduous task. Sometimes, the hurdles appear too numerous or too high. Other times, the resources are too scarce, the time in a day too short, and the willingness of others to do the morally obvious right thing nonexistent. For these ailments, I wish I could offer a cure that wasn't solely based on dogged persistence. Unfortunately, this is the stark reality, particularly in a time when our elected officials have left us in—what the editorial board of the New England Journal of Medicine calls—a "leadership vacuum." As of October 30, 2020, there have been nearly 230,000 deaths from COVID-19 with no end in sight.

In Milwaukee County, the key pandemic safety indicators have rapidly changed from green to yellow to red while, at the same time, homicides in 2020 have surpassed the previous record of 174 set in 1993, and reached 189 by the end of the year. Structural racism is rampant, and, as I mentioned previously, the infant mortality rate in Milwaukee is among the worst in the nation. And as if that is not enough, MCW has lost another medical student to suicide—one of our immediate family. We can't even protect ourselves, and if this doesn't give us all pause and insight into our failures, it is entirely unclear to me what will.

We clearly need a curriculum and culture dedicated to medical student and clinician well-being, public health, advocacy, legislation, and community engagement so we can train tomorrow's doctors to work within these spheres and remain healthy while doing so.

———————————

There should not have existed the need for us, as a grassroots group at a medical school, to take on the task of widespread and concise public health messaging about voter safety and empowerment. Yet, as the pandemic rages on and in the midst of a leadership vacuum, we did what we could. We are proud of our efforts, have learned from them, and will continue to work tirelessly with this growing knowledge for the betterment of those in our communities.

RBG and Dad

Adina Kalet, MD MPH

As the country was mourning the death of Ruth Bader GInsburg in September 2020, Dr. Kalet was being vigilant to her father's needs as he navigated a health crisis. In this essay, she shared how Justice Ginsburg's visionary thinking and vigilance empowered women to be decision makers and leaders with a "place at the table."

This week, the death of Justice Ruth Bader Ginsburg has been on my mind. I realized how important she has been to us. I have benefited from, and been moved by, her critical and prophetic message that, "Women belong in all places where decisions are being made." For women of my generation, this was not the norm and it is still far from a guarantee. Thanks to the work of RBG and a handful of others, some of us now find ourselves "at the table," making decisions and expanding our spheres of influence as we attempt to make the world a better place. Her work led directly to transformative change. Many of us who would have otherwise been sidelined are now heard in ways that would never have been possible without her.

Ruth Bader Ginsburg was an American hero and transformational leader, *par excellence*. People on all points of the political spectrum noted her uncanny ability to listen, her impact on society, her brilliance and courage, her prophetic legal mind, her ability to see things as they should be for all people, and her perseverance. I have medical colleagues who take on the challenges inherent in medicine the same way.

This week, the chance to be heard became personal.

I am writing this column while sitting in a hospital waiting room, the daughter of someone suddenly thrust into the medical system. In my new unwelcome role, I feel vulnerable and less assured of the value of my personal "power and influence." I had planned to write about RBG's life and legacy. Instead, I find myself searching for parallels between how she leveraged her knowledge of the legal system for change and my need to exercise my familiarity with the medical system to make certain my father stays safe. Like her, I remain vigilant, paying attention to everything that is happening around us, and advocating on my father's behalf. It can be exhausting.

My dad is a remarkably fit eighty-four-year-old retired engineer who presented this past Tuesday to his internist with classic symptoms of exertional angina in a crescendo pattern. Dad's EKG had developed nonspecific T-waves that suggested something amiss. He was walked down the hall to the cardiologist who then called the interventional cardiologist who scheduled a cardiac catheterization. He was admitted to the ER for monitoring. His first troponin levels (an indicator of heart muscle cell damage) were equivocal, suggesting heart muscle cells were spilling their contents, but he didn't appear to be having a full-blown heart attack.

For context, my dad sees a doctor in the large academic medical center where I did my residency training and spent the first thirty years of my career. I know this place and these people—warts, glory, and all. Even though I had confidence in his care team, I was terrified. I knew too much. I never left his side because, over the years, I have seen all of the things that can go wrong even when everyone is well-meaning and highly qualified.

From the patient's (and the daughter's) perspective, hospital care separates individuals from everything familiar. There are endless streams of humans with uncertain duties, repeated handoffs between nurses, physicians, and other staff, long (ten-hour!) waits in the ER until a "clean bed" becomes available, no proffered food, malfunctioning cardiac monitors for a patient with a heart problem, a mix of disturbingly poor and remarkably skillful communications, and moments of caring and compassion juxtaposed with moments of "ghosting." Even as someone who knows medicine and trained in the hospital where we now sat, the experience was dehumanizing.

Further, I could see the contrast between the technical, sophisticated wonders of modern medicine—cardiac catheterization suites with cutting-edge technology and physicians with impeccable expertise—and the troubling implications of the corporate commodification of healing in healthcare systems. Some patients in the city are offered luxurious private rooms with gourmet meals and spectacular views of the river while others— in the public hospital down the street—are offered no amenities. The public hospital's professional expertise is, fortunately, comparable, but is also distinguished by the staff's ability to offer excellent care despite their lack of resources.

What's the bigger picture here? How might we make healthcare more equitable? RBG had a wider vision of society, and she pushed the legal system to treat everyone equally no matter their gender or status. In the same way, visionaries in medicine envision a future where every person is entitled to safe, high quality, compassionate, cost-effective healthcare. We must include the most vulnerable patients, even as she fiercely advocated for all members of society. We will face challenges along the way, just as she experienced blatant interpersonal and institutional sexism during her career.

She demonstrated that, to be transformational, we need to be persistent. There was a moment, early in her time at Harvard, when RGB and her small group of women classmates were challenged by the law school dean to defend why they "took" men's spots in law school. They demonstrated their value with their actions and dedication. They showed that they belonged. Later, despite graduating at the top of her class and being part of the law review, she could not get a clerkship or even a job with a law firm. She chose an alternative path, doing comparative international law research, joining a law school faculty, and creating her own way forward. She ended up changing the world.

To achieve transformation, we will need to engage—like RBG did—in necessary, nuanced, and difficult conversations. She had a clear moral compass. She was able to change her mind, to be influenced by others, and to learn deep and abiding truths about human dignity from those whom she loved and especially from those she didn't know. With these character traits, it is possible to engage in respectful, caring, civically responsible, and sometimes fierce dialogues on contentious issues, including the inequities in healthcare and society.

"You can disagree without being disagreeable," she said. "Fight for the things that you care about but do it in a way that will lead others to join you." Although being patient enough to work through issues can be a huge challenge, her long view of history allowed her to dissent while remaining part of rich, mutually respectful, humble relationships with those with whom she fundamentally disagreed. Her ability to persuade without fracturing human connections is one of her most important legacies and lessons.

I accompanied my dad on his journey this week. Happily, he had the best possible care and had a wonderful outcome despite the frightening situation. I advocated for him, speaking up and influencing the system when it faltered. But mostly, we realized that the outcome was a result of the fundamental commitment of his medical professionals to care for someone in need.

RBG, too, depended largely on the goodness of people working in the legal system, although she did not allow that faith to keep her from being a vigilant advocate when she felt it was needed. She believed in the goodness of others, but also that she had the responsibility to drive the change. She persisted, and the world is a better place because of it. May we all be inspired by her courage and passion.

Being Human in Medicine:
We Are Fabulous Failures

Himanshu Agrawal, MD

In this essay about dealing with stigma, Dr. Agrawal shared his own story of hopelessness and reminded readers that failure is not the same as defeat.

It's 2:00 am, and I am a junior medical student in India. I haven't eaten in two days and am worsening my heartburn—and my heartbreak—with black coffee and a cigarette. I can feel the sense of doom grip my fundus. A senior medical student whom I barely know staggers into the cafeteria, happy to have a brief respite from his overnight rotation. "Why the long face?" he asks out of genuine concern.

The tears erupt, uninvited. "I did horrible in my USMLE Step 1 exam!" I tell him. I hardly know the guy, but I am in mourning, so shame be damned.

"There, there! It can't be that bad. How much did you score?"

Envisioning my entire future evaporating in front of me, I manage to say the numbers: "197."

The man takes a step back, and his hand instinctively rises to stroke his chin. It's as if he has heard someone mutter a terminal diagnosis. "Hmm . . . That is bad! Well . . . with a score like that, you won't be able to get into internal medicine . . . the only US residency you can get into is psychiatry . . ."

Suddenly, he meets a reaction he likely did not expect. A wide grin appears on my tear-smudged face. "Really?! But that's what I want to do! Psychiatry!"

He looks at me with surprise, then smiles. "Well then what are you crying for? Let's celebrate! This cup of tea is on you, my friend!"

The year was 2000. Psychiatry was not nearly as competitive as it is now, and international medical graduates still got interviews in American programs. Much has changed in the last twenty years, but some things remain the same. You see, looking back, this random stranger had no idea what he was talking about—he was certainly no authority on USMLE scores, successes, and failures—but, like so many others, he was a speculation-guru, a pundit of pontification. Unknowingly, his prophesying was exactly the piece of straw I needed to stay afloat!

Hopelessness cast as large a shadow on me back

then as it has, over the years, for several of my medical students. And sometimes, it is as quickly dispelled as mine was that fateful day by that clueless senior student (sometimes it takes a bit longer).

I am writing today for all my students who have recently faced despair or who may one day be met with crippling news. This Distinguished Fellow of the American Psychiatric Association, this latest recipient of Edward J. Lennon Endowed Clinical Teaching Award, this boy from New Delhi who grew up without running water but who now swims in a 29,000-gallon swimming pool (feel free to insert your own yardstick of success), I was once ready to walk away from it all. I was ready to throw in the towel.

I am so glad I didn't.

Remember two things. Firstly, you are not as good as they say you are when you succeed, and you are never as bad as they say you are when you fail. Secondly, you will never cherish success more sweetly, than when you have had to swallow the bitterness of failure.

Do I wish you failure? Of course not. What I am saying is this: there is more to life, *so much more*, after failure. Failure is not the same as defeat.

They say nothing succeeds like success. They have not seen the daily grin on the face of this Fabulous Failure.

A Thanksgiving Reflection

Karen Marcdante, MD

At Thanksgiving 2020, Dr. Marcdante gave thanks for the people who bring light to the world, even as we might grieve their passing.

"At times, our own light goes out and is rekindled by a spark from another person. Each of us has cause to think with deep gratitude of those who have lighted the flame within us."
—Albert Schweitzer

These days, it seems that there are lots of lights to be rekindled. Who knew that our lives would change so much due to a microscopic organism? I don't know about you, but I have recognized that I am grieving the loss of our former lives. It is the little things. I miss the drive to and from work, when I had a chance to plan and reflect on my day. I really, really miss, terribly, those moments in the hallways when I passed colleagues. Whether it was a smile and a quick hello or stopping the other person for a quick chat or some problem-solving, those moments of connection were there, but they now no longer occur without planning. Acknowledging that I am, in fact, grieving is a good first step. And recognizing that it was grief resulted in returning to a time when I grieved the most.

I was seventeen when, early one morning, the phone rang. My dad answered, then hit a wall with his fist. My mom had just died after a short battle with an unknown cancer. The lights went out for my dad, my sisters, and me. Fortunately, we had many who helped us to rekindle that light. I have realized that my mom, even in her absence, was also involved in relighting and maintaining that light. As we work to have character development become an explicit part of our curriculum at MCW, I realize just how important role models who demonstrated their character strengths daily (such as my mom) can be.

My mom was an amazing woman. She went to Marquette School of Nursing at a time when women most often stayed home. She gave birth to and raised my five sisters and me, working full-time to make ends meet. As a nurse, she worked third shift until we were all in school for a full day. Then, she went back to school, gaining the credentials she needed to become a public health nurse. She had a quiet, strong faith, a tomboy's love of sports, and a wicked sense of humor. It is with deep gratitude that I think about all I did learn from her: that kindness is the key to building relationships; that following your heart brings you success, even through the many challenges; that persistence augments any of your natural abilities and can help you as you strive for excellence; that humor (or the well-aimed glass of water during a spontaneous water fight at the dinner table) brings people together with zest and joy. While I may not have recognized it when I was younger, I also recognize that she had amazing patience, hope, and a spirituality that rose above the differences in religions in which my parents were raised. She encouraged us all to be curious and to be strong, independent women. When she faced her death at a very early age, she chose to exhibit bravery, grace, and gratitude.

Since those days, I have been blessed to have many other strong role models in my life, each exhibiting character strengths that have helped make the world a better place. I am grateful for each and every one of them. Mentors and colleagues alike have provided kindness, love and, let's face it, the prudence I needed as I faced challenges. The many learners with whom I have been honored to work often infuse my life with their bravery (it's hard to be a medical student!), zest, curiosity, and perspectives. They remind me every day that life is full of opportunities if you look for them.

And in this day, when I grieve about the differences in my daily activities, I am grateful that these people are still here, persevering under conditions that are new to us all. There is so much to be grateful for! This Thanksgiving, I will pray that they all stay happy and healthy and are blessed with others who offer a helping hand, an open mind, and a kind word.

Our world is certainly challenging the lights in our life but, gratefully, our world is also full of people who can rekindle them. Be safe!

A Medical Student's Remorse | My Anatomy Group

Hayden Swartz

*This is an original poem by MCW-Green Bay
medical student Hayden Swartz.*

I struggled with disassembly at first,
I was the most comfortable in my group, however.

I was assigned
Difficult
Uncomfortable
Maneuvers.

I did not mind the harder tasks.

I started to be intrigued.
I started to be numb.

When others grimace
I feel nothing.

I am a germaphobe
And yet I feel okay.

What would my mother say?

Community Reflections: What has been the best part of your day today?

An anonymous reader submitted this response:

Waking up remembering that women can be elected to work in the White House!!!

Community Reflections: What quote has been on your mind lately?

Brittany Player, DO submitted this response:

"Courage doesn't always roar. Sometimes courage is the little voice at the end of the day that says, 'I'll try again tomorrow.'"

—Mary Anne Radmacher

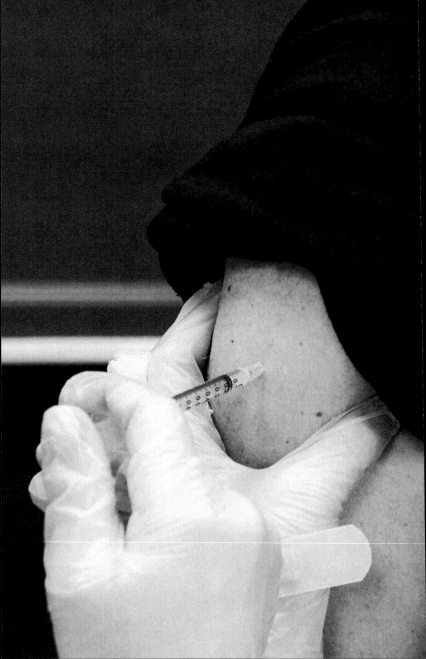

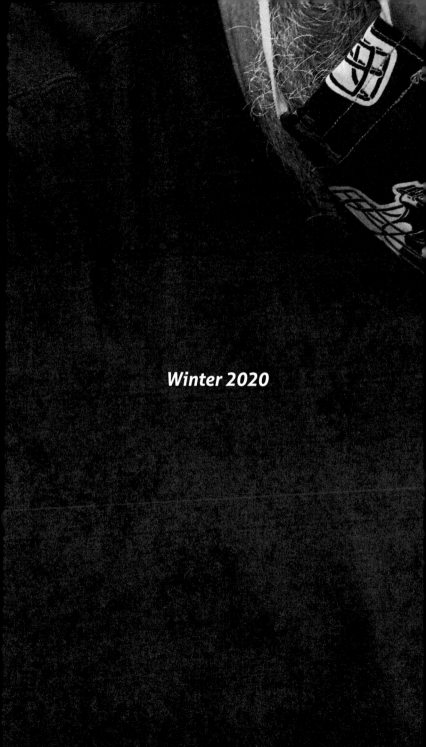

Winter 2020

A Turn of the Clock: A Student Perspective on Remaining "Present" in Medical School

Chase LaRue

Several months into the pandemic, Mr. LaRue, an MCW-Milwaukee medical student, reflected on how he was adapting to the new reality by "doing less" and managing his time and attention.

Tuesday morning. 9:46 am. I've been awake for five hours, but I still have two more hours of lectures to watch. A mid-morning nap teases me from the bed just a few feet behind me. Snacks are within grasp if only I . . . uh . . . *Lecture! Cardiovascular pathology! Lecture, Chase, Lecture!*

This internal conversation has been common since mid-March. Like many at MCW and the Kern Institute, my life took on dramatic changes when my normal study location was ripped from underneath me. Medical school, relationships, and my well-being shifted as quickly as the hands on a clock face.

Whenever I sat down to do something, rather than focusing on what needed to be done, I was distracted. Think about that friend who is always on their phone, even when you are speaking right to them. It doesn't feel great, and you don't get the feeling they "care" about you. That was what I was doing to myself. It's me. I'm the friend to myself. I've figuratively been on my phone rather than giving each moment a full look. Both in school and in life.

When I came to medical school, I knew exactly what I hoped to build for myself while embodying the student-doctor persona. The pandemic hasn't changed my pursuit; rather, it has provided detours and scenic views that I did not have in my original blueprint.

So, you wonder, "What did Chase envision for medical school?" Despite the risk of oversimplifying the learning experience, I'll summarize my hopes and my commitment in a few short words: investment, purpose, and present-ness. And though my attention disorder doesn't necessarily enhance these hopes, it does ride shotgun to the COVID-19 that is driving my M2 year.

I don't know what these goals look like for anyone else, but here is how they look to me.

Investment

Medical students are a unique brand of learners. We willingly invest at least eleven years of our lives just to claim the "attending physician" title. When we don the white coat or make that first cadaveric incision, our souls reignite with a sense of "this is how I get there," and few feelings will ever replace that. I am no different. I pride myself on a "jump in headfirst" type of commitment.

But when most of the doctor-like learning environment was taken from me, my commitment to the investment was challenged and, honestly, broke down. The big picture became full of telehealth and recorded lectures. I didn't like it. Suddenly, I craved the frigid temperatures of MCW's Kerrigan Auditorium just to recall how uncomfortable it could be to willingly pursue the dream.

And then it hits me. This pandemic is nothing but a speed bump in my education. *How might I double down and reinvest my energy?* Medical school is hard, but I knew that "challenge" was nonnegotiable in this process. I reinvested. I sat down with my journal, and revisited why I gave up another career to someday be a physician.

Purpose

Sick kids, sad families, and my own memories of emergency room waiting rooms brought me here. My experience with health disparities pushed me, and my sense of belonging while working in a clinic got me up in the morning. But when my Clinical Apprenticeship rotation was restricted in 2020, my ability to connect with my education shifted; people are my purpose, health is my outcome. *Where are they now? Why am I still here? How can I keep caring?* I search my work for the places where I can continue to connect with my purpose.

Present-ness

The crux of medical education—of every patient encounter, the attention to detail required for high quality care—is in every moment. The more I felt cheated by circumstances, the more I realized I was missing the bigger picture. Despite the challenges set forth by these "unprecedented times," I remembered something that I was asked the first time I stepped on a baseball field as a teenager. My coach challenged me then with, "What are you going to get out of this moment? This practice?"

I thought of my coach as I reread my personal statement for medical school and looked over my interview notes. I remembered one important fact: MCW has my academic trust, that's why I came here. MCW trusts me to work within my means to grow into a capable student-doctor. I realized I had shifted my focus to drama, excuses, and self-deprecation. I believed I was absorbed in my education when I was, instead, overwhelmed by the stimuli around me.

And so, I reassessed my purpose and my investment in the journey. I asked myself what I needed to do to be "present" in my learning, my relationships, and my goals. The answer surprised me. It was, *Do less.*

Do less?

Before the pandemic, I had struggled for hours under the assumption that "more is better," and when my office and bedroom became the same place, it was even easier to let work and life become the same thing. It never worked out for me.

My solution? A thirty-minute hourglass where I

dedicate one turn to one activity and one activity only. If I finish early, I take a break. If I need more time, I note my progress, take a five-minute break and start fresh with another turn. Whether it's a small group (where I still take a break to disconnect after thirty minutes), a lecture, or this article, staying present in the pandemic requires struggle and suffering, but my thirty-minute intervals offer a soft reminder of why I'm here and provide the attention the work deserves. Just as we have windows of time set aside for patients, meetings, or other tasks, I use my hourglass method to fully commit myself to each moment.

This approach has brought me back. My hourglass has made me pay attention to the present and helped me make each moment one of commitment.

Looking for a Leader?
You've Got the Wrong Person

Mario Castellanos

In this essay on leadership, Mario Castellanos, a native of Honduras and MCW-Milwaukee medical student, shared his discovery that serving others as a tutor helped him grow in ways he did not anticipate.

Until a few years ago, the title of this article was a reality for me. I used to not see myself as a leader. In fact, sometimes I still have trouble seeing myself as one. Growing up in Honduras, I only perceived those in public office or the managerial positions of the business world as "leaders." My primary and secondary education didn't particularly emphasize leadership as an essential attribute of any other budding professional. It would take moving to the US to realize that I, too, could become a leader.

After moving to the United States for college, I

ventured into leadership activities as a way to maximize the benefits of my American education. My plan (and lifelong dream) was to become a physician in the US, so I knew I needed to stand out somehow. It also seemed that many of my peers placed a large amount of value on "being a leader," and many people talked about taking leadership positions in campus organizations; it was what the cool kids did. As an impressionable foreign student, I followed suit.

Little by little, I began joining different organizations on campus. The intent was to rise up the ranks and eventually hold a position on the executive board. In my view at the time, to be a leader, I had to hold a position of significant influence in the group. I won't bore you with the details, but I was unable to ever hold a presidency or similar position in any of my organizations during college. I always perceived that as a personal failure, and I graduated college thinking that leadership just wasn't meant for me.

The opportunity to tutor

Fast forward a few years, I was a medical student at MCW. I had a clean slate to reconstruct myself for the next four years. This time, I was no longer a newbie. I had grown accustomed to the educational system and developed much-needed confidence. Just as in college, I began pursuing my interests through membership in student organizations with the hopes of aspiring to leadership positions within them.

However, in contrast to college, I discovered two new activities: education and mentorship. I've been privileged to be a student tutor for the last three years of medical school. As a tutor, I'm in charge of facilitating course and medical boards material. I meet with my peers one-on one or in small groups to answer their questions and deliver review sessions.

Little did I know that these experiences would completely change my view of leadership.

When I applied for employment as a tutor, I never expected it to be one of the most defining experiences of my medical school career. I never anticipated the connections I would build with my peers across all years or how my duties would transcend beyond tutoring. Fairly soon, the focus of my sessions pivoted from solely teaching to also mentoring. In all of my tutoring sessions, I make it a priority to check on my peers and act as a resource for them to be successful in medical school. I strive to encourage and support those around me to become the best version of themselves.

Lessons learned

One of the most important lessons I have gained from tutoring is that leadership can be practiced anywhere, from a business meeting to a casual session on how to do well in a class. Being an educator and mentor requires a great deal of motivation, listening skills, empathy, and self-awareness, all necessary attributes of a good leader. A leader is someone who creates meaningful bonds with individuals and invests in the development of others. As a tutor, I've had the privilege of developing those traits and derived great joy from the connections with my peers. In a way, being a tutor makes me a leader.

Throughout the residency application season, I often get asked about my most meaningful leadership experience. Invariably, my answer always is being a tutor. If you had asked me to predict the answer as a first-year medical student, I would've imagined being president of a major campus organization. How differently things turned out. Along the way, I learned that one doesn't need a glamorous title or to deliver magnificent speeches to qualify as a leader; being a leader starts within, and sometimes all you need is the willingness to connect with individuals and make a positive impact on the lives of others.

The "Ethics of Care": What Does That Look Like?

Adina Kalet MD MPH

In this essay, Dr. Kalet shared the story of a friend whose surgical procedure left her suffering and whose surgeon left her feeling alone. She wondered, what does true caring look like?

A good friend of mine is suffering. She recently underwent what is typically a relatively straightforward surgical procedure both she and her physician expected would correct a disabling problem and improve her quality of life. Instead, she developed a rare, perplexing, painful complication that significantly limits her mobility, interferes with getting a good night's sleep, and has not responded well to treatments. And she essentially has been abandoned by the surgeon who performed the procedure.

When, months later, it became clear that she was not

going to recover as expected, the surgeon ultimately made a general referral to see a pain specialist and only referred her to physical therapy on the patient's request. He does see her in "follow-up" but focuses only on the immediate post-operative issues, not the new condition. When my friend reaches out to inform him of her progress and asks clarifying questions or for advice, the registered nurse on his team responds to her messages in a curt "just the facts," perfunctory manner. For a few months post-surgery, the office reached out to inquire about her progress through an imprecise and impersonal "app," though no one has expressed care or concern that her pain continues. In my book, this is abandonment and, therefore, unethical.

An obligation and responsibility to care

As physicians, we have both an obligation and responsibility to care for, with, and about our patients. Like other service providers, we have a "duty of care," which is a legal obligation requiring us to adhere to "standards of reasonable care while performing any acts that could foreseeably harm others." From this perspective, strictly speaking, my friend's surgeon did his duty. And given the current fragmentation of healthcare into sub-specialties, he can argue that by ensuring postoperative wound healing, he is discharging his obligations. But this is not caring.

The "Ethics of Care," developed by feminist scholars Carol Gilligan and Joan Tronto among many others, holds that moral action goes beyond meeting standards—being objective and justice-orientated—and centers on the relationships and connection with others, especially when they are vulnerable and require expertise. The Ethics of Care emphasizes the importance of attentiveness and responsiveness to the individual, and acknowledges the complexity of caretaking. Rather than taking a narrow view on the obligation to refer my friend to a competent expert, I believe this physician had a responsibility to do the complex, skilled work of caring for her. He demonstrated no intention to do anything beyond his narrowly focused area of expertise.

When I told my friend's story to a mentor who is an experienced surgeon, he said, *"These are the patients you hold close, you give them your personal cell phone number, you respond and see them often until there is some resolution or even if there isn't one. You are in this relationship for the long haul."* The wise and ethical physician makes the referrals, ensures the patient understands what needs to be done, has the difficult conversations, and "quarterbacks" the game until there is a resolution.

By any measure, my friend is a "good" patient. She takes medication as prescribed, engages in physical therapy with enthusiasm and commitment, listens carefully to the recommendations and advice of her physician, engages actively in decision-making, and is extremely well informed. Luckily, she has a caring pain management specialist and access to friends and relatives who are in healthcare. I have advised her to move on and consider the surgeon who operated on her as she would any highly paid tradesman rather than as her physician. This is terribly disappointing, but common.

True caring seeks to relieve suffering, especially when the going gets tough

To be clear, while this isn't likely "malpractice," it is, in my view, clinical incompetence. My friend's current predicament was not due to a mistake in judgement or poor surgical technique, but her physician did not take responsibility to relieve her suffering by actively, assertively, compassionately, and competently *caring for her*. To do this well, he would have needed a mature, internalized professional identity to help him make morally-informed choices in a therapeutic and caring relationship, especially when things got frustrating or went wrong. It would enable him to spend the time and make the effort to communicate with this patient directly, guide her to effective symptom relief and sincerely empathize with her situation. This is not easy—sophisticated clinical communication skills are required. These include being capable of actively listening, while accurately identifying and appropriately responding to emotions, all while conducting clinical reasoning and creative problem-solving. These are learnable skills but require both desire and practice to master. This physician is not trying hard enough.

All physicians need to take responsibility for caring for patients, *especially* when the going gets tough, vexing, perplexing, and challenging, like when a patient who should have recovered does not. In one way or another, managing chronic pain is the responsibility of all physicians. Central to effective pain control, from the patient's point of view, is being taken seriously, remaining hopeful and realistic, being listened to, and experiencing authentic empathy from a trustworthy physician or other healthcare professional. Anyone who has gone through childbirth understands that extreme pain—as long as it is going to be time-limited and will end with the birth of a healthy infant—can be "suffered" without medication, be well-tolerated, and can even be experienced as joyful when surrounded by trustworthy, caring, and competent health professionals. On the flip side, even mild to moderate pain can be unbearable when "suffered" alone or is a sign of loss of bodily integrity, increasing disability, or a terminal diagnosis. A mature and skillful physician has the potential to relieve suffering simply by staying in the relationship with the patient.

Modern medicine takes place within complex institutions and, even with the best intentions, the incentives can be perverse. If care and caring must happen within trustworthy relationships, then healthcare systems that divide the labor so that everyone works at the "top of their license" are dividing the patient. I worry that as a side effect of "team care," healthcare professionals are being encouraged, incentivized, or forced to destroy therapeutic relationships. This is why physicians must have a strong character and a moral compass, a sense of agency, and masterful communication skills to remain "the patient's doctor" when there is rough going—staying put when it would be more comfortable to leave or send in someone else.

I have spent much of my career learning, teaching, and studying patient-physician communications. To motivate others to take this very seriously, I often point out that patients are more likely to sue a physician for "abandonment" of the type described here than for actual malpractice. People will, I believe, forgive mistakes but not a lack of care.

Walking with Purpose at Sixty-Four

Sandra Pfister, PhD

Dr. Pfister, a cardiovascular pharmacologist and foundational sciences course director, wrote about how the pandemic challenged her to reexamine her purpose as a teacher, a scientist, and as a person.

I turned sixty-four in January 2020: the year of COVID-19. It's not surprising then that John Lennon and Paul McCartney's lyrics, "Will you still need me, will you still feed me, when I'm sixty-four," have started to resonate with me more and more these days. It doesn't help that there have been a few misplaced words from some of our politicians that older people would (should) risk death in order to keep the economy open during the crisis.

I often tell myself that I'm "not that old," but the daily video conferences where I get to see my face up-close-and-personal on my computer screen keep reminding me otherwise. In addition to trying to find settings that allow me to touch-up my image, I have thought maybe I should wear makeup while working from home, something I rarely do when at work.

Yet, it's not really about the number of years behind me or the wrinkles I see on the screen, but more about the words of Lennon and McCartney. It's about wondering whether I am needed in this time of COVID-19. I will never be a frontline caregiver. My training as a vascular pharmacologist is unlikely to make me an essential worker. Will you still need me when I'm sixty-four?

Like many, my days are not spent doing what I was trained to do. My lab is in hibernation. While I anticipated this would free me to finish a manuscript and design experiments for a new grant submission, these things have not yet happened.

I am a course director for M1 Principles of Drug Action Course. With COVID-19, the course changes have been fairly straightforward, but the "extras" have taken time and energy. We transitioned our traditional paper-and-pencil, short answer and fill in the blank exams to multiple choice questions on a computer. Not so easy.

I also worry about the isolation of our M1s, and I struggle with ways to keep myself and the other faculty connected to them. I feel a constant need to answer every email I receive from a student as soon as possible. Not so easy.

Since I no longer commute to work, I don't have that car time to play my motivational music for the day. For unknown reasons, I find myself starting my workday long before I did in the office. I wonder if I am attempting to convince myself that my work is valuable. Will you still need me when I'm sixty-four?

Recognizing that I will not live forever, I have begun to think about this process in a different way. It has ended up being a good time for me to reflect and remind myself that I chose my path to be a basic science researcher for a purpose. And that purpose continues to exist even as others might see aging people as less useful or, as I have sensed, less valuable during the pandemic.

As Charles Dickens wrote, *"The best way to lengthen out our days is to walk steadily and with a purpose."* I haven't figured out this new reality of life in the time of COVID-19, but I am getting better at convincing myself that my sense of purpose never really changed. My life was purposeful before COVID-19, it remains purposeful during COVID-19, and will continue to be purposeful long after COVID-19 is over. I will continue to walk steadily and answer affirmatively that, yes, you will still need me when I'm sixty-four.

Anonymity and the Shape of a Soul

Jake Taxis, MDiv BCC

With COVID-19 face-to-face visiting restrictions in place, Pastor Taxis, one of the hospital chaplains, found that he was able to connect in important ways with patients even when all they could share was their voices.

In the beginning of her poem, "Some Questions You Might Ask," Mary Oliver finds herself reflecting on the soul:

Is the soul solid, like iron?
Or is it tender and breakable,
like the wings of a moth in the beak of the owl?
Who has it, and who doesn't? . . .
Does it have a shape? Like an iceberg?
Like the eye of a hummingbird?

This poem haunts me for a few reasons, not least of which because, as a palliative care chaplain and Lutheran minister, I listen to the souls of people every day. That is an odd thing to say, I know, and not a little pretentious.

But, chaplain or not, we all find ourselves, sometimes unexpectedly, listening to the *souls* of others, souls with very different *shapes*. Raw authenticity can break the surface of any conversation without warning, especially in a hospital room, and instead of a dreary verbal cliché, we hear a *soul*.

There are those moments when a patient's soul seems disarmingly "tender and breakable, like the wings of a moth," and others which almost appear as icebergs, cold and coarse, understandably angry at whatever authored the terrible circumstances in which they find themselves.

The shape of one's soul

Few signs point to the shape of one's soul more directly than one's physicality, particularly the eyes. One cannot help but remember the observation of a first century Nazarene rabbi, who had something to say about that: "The eye is the lamp of the body . . ."

So much is communicated by a patient's posture and physical space. Some patient rooms are nothing if not temporary archives, filled with photographs of a life lived outside of this impersonal, sterilized cube. Drawings from grandchildren, flowers from a sister in California, a letter of encouragement from a former coworker. All of it has something to say about the human being lying in that bed, and the shape his soul has taken over the many years preceding this illness.

Being an "anonymous" chaplain during COVID-19 restrictions

Physical presentation matters when it comes to navigating the soul of another, and so, when chaplains were asked to begin making phone calls to patients on certain units, rather than seeing them in person, I was more than a little disappointed. What good would a disembodied voice over a telephone do for a patient when such rich and comforting communication is delivered nonverbally? And then, the personal doubts: Could I respond compassionately and carefully to the particular shape of a soul over a phone—especially when the only information I would have is the tone of a voice from some faraway corner of the hospital?

One of the strange things I learned early on as a chaplain is that patients are often quite eager and even more willing to speak with a chaplain than with their own pastor, priest, or rabbi. People like anonymity, and no one is more anonymous than a chaplain: You may see us once during your hospitalization, at which point you pour out your heart, and never see us again. You see your pastor every Sunday, and God only knows what you might have told her while medicated. That's a good recipe for awkward—particularly during the next church potluck. Chaplains are safe, at least in part, because they are anonymous.

Here lies the remarkable treasure upon which I stumbled while calling patients over the phone, especially those who were COVID-19 positive. Without question, I missed the communicative possibilities of physical presence with a patient. And yet, I could not ignore the unexpected return I received on the simple investment of dialing a number and embracing, if only for a few moments, the role of *anonymous* pastor. I really didn't know these patients, and they really didn't know me—but we found a shared language of belief by voice alone, and that made all the difference.

In some cases, our shared anonymity (and the patient's newfound vulnerability) partnered to form some weirdly wonderful moments: like the patient who shared, in vibrant detail, about an angelic visitation she experienced earlier in life; the longtime truck driver whose preference for being alone fit nicely with the solitude of his hospital room; or the patient whose remarks on her dinner gave us both a good laugh before we prayed together. "People with this virus are fighting for their lives . . . Give them something to look forward to, something that at least *looks* fresh," she laughed.

That is not to say our conversations were not also deeply emotional and, more often than not, terribly sad. One's longing for a sense of God's presence—or any semblance of meaning—in the midst of medical uncertainty is not limited to one kind of patient. Souls, I have learned, take on very different shapes at different times.

When your only source of information is a voice, listening deeply (and differently) is not only necessary, it's primary. One of the differences is an absence of the physical self. The space you share with a patient is constricted (physical cues are removed), but it is also expanded (you can almost entirely get out of the way). You are a voice on the other end of the phone, and for most of the call, you're likely silent. Your physical presence is not doing what it normally does, sending subtle cues that may or may not be taken the right way.

True listeners . . . are free to receive, welcome, and accept

These moments of shared anonymity over the phone felt more to me like eavesdropping on a prayer then engaging in pastoral counseling. Therein lies the beauty. If one is willing to step aside, anonymity can cultivate an open space for deeper disclosure and care.

The late Catholic priest, philosopher, and theologian Henri Nouwen had much to say about a kind of listening that is liberated from normal social tendencies:

> *To listen is very hard, because it asks of us so much interior stability that we no longer need to prove ourselves by speeches, arguments, statements or declarations. True listeners no longer have an inner need to make their presence known. They are free to receive, welcome, to accept.*

Listening to a soul is more than hearing words. It's about freeing up space and learning to be, if only for a moment, anonymous. There is a strange and wonderful glory in two people talking over a hospital phone, unmarred by self-assertion and agenda. Ironically, anonymity can actually become the way to authentic rapport and understanding. The shape of the soul becomes visible when we get out of one another's way.

Egalitarian, Loving Relationships and Career Satisfaction

Adina Kalet, MD MPH

In this essay from Valentine's Day 2021, Dr. Kalet reviewed data that showed physicians in "egalitarian" relationships experienced greater career satisfaction. How might medical and resident education support and nurture these important human connections?

Translational researchers save lives, but over 40% of physician-scientists leave academic medicine. COVID-19 has highlighted the importance of having these types of investigators engaged and on the ground to lead the charge to discovery while caring for both patients and populations. They are best positioned to detect emerging disease variants, run innovative therapeutic trials, and move new discoveries from the bench to the bedside and into the community. We also count on them to train the next generation of physician-scientists.

The departure of active physician-scientists causes a serious shortage of researchers and a huge loss to the health science workforce. Given how exciting and important their work is, why do so many step off the track?

I believe they leave because of the constant and recurring challenges these individuals face trying to balance their own lives while attempting to pursue meaningful clinical and research careers. Without solid, deep, and meaningful support both at home and at work, the challenging lives of clinician-scientists can become overwhelming.

What does this have to do with Valentine's Day?

In our recent paper entitled "Challenges, Joys, and Career Satisfaction of Women Graduates of the Robert Wood Johnson Clinical Scholars Program 1973–2011," our group, including Dr. Kathlyn Fletcher, reported on a long-term study of the women graduates of this highly successful fellowship aimed at training change agents in the transformation of American healthcare quality. Among many findings, we identified that—of all these remarkably successful and influential women—the most satisfied were likely to describe their work as ". . . deeply meaningful and have egalitarian spousal relationships." The views of these well-trained women clinician-scientists offer important lessons to those interested in repairing the leaky pipeline of clinical researchers.

Most of the program graduates in our study were in committed, dual-career, personal partnerships. What did "egalitarian spousal relationships" mean to them? It was very complex. We asked the women, some younger and some close to retirement, to reflect on the course of their working lives. On one hand, successful respondents noted that culturally determined and structurally maintained "traditional" gender social roles became flexible and negotiated over time as the needs of the couple changed. A small number of the women in our study reported that, during the child rearing stage of their lives, their partners were the primary parents while they were the sole employed spouse. Most women, though, were constantly juggling home and work. While some respondents reported satisfying lives of "serial monogamy," divorce was uniformly reported as disruptive to careers and life satisfaction.

Even as they support early career clinical investigators and scientists, funders such as the National Institutes of Health, the Robert Wood Johnson Foundation, and the Doris Duke Charitable Foundation have not explicitly and formally addressed how to create, maintain, and sustain "egalitarian spousal relationships" that might be associated with a thriving, impactful, and flourishing life in medicine and science. This might be an area for future study.

What would a relationship curriculum for clinician scientists (and others) cover?

Love relationships, although universally seen as positive and important, are typically firmly in the personal and private domain. Most of us learn how to make a life from our own families, our particular cultural groups, or our close peers. Career-focused women in my generation, facing lives very different from that of our parents, had to be creative. We talked "offline" with our peers, scanned our mentors' offices for evidence of outside lives (e.g., family photos, children's artwork, dry cleaning, grocery lists), and asked directly when it seemed safe: *"How do you do it all?" "Who does the laundry?" "When the kids are sick, who stays home?" "When do the grants get written?" "How do you decide if it is right to relocate?"*

When I was raising my own children, I loved gently interrogating medical students and residents who had "working mothers." I asked about their experiences and views, hoping to learn anything that would improve my chance of being a good mother. Since then, there has been an accumulation of material to read and discuss. Role models are more common. We can now think about what a structured curriculum might include.

There is much to learn about finding love, building healthy relationships, and negotiating lives of meaning while not driving each other crazy! When I was starting out, it would have been great to have access to "paired" autobiographies, such as Michele Obama's *Becoming* and Barack Obama's *A Promised Land*, to gain insight from each partner's point of view into how hard, but inspiring, it is to maintain a loving relationship under the pressures of "dueling" careers. We can learn from others as they cope with the types of accumulated, complex life experiences that author Nikos Kazantzakis had his protagonist Zorba the Greek lament when he said, *"I'm a man, so I'm married. Wife, children, house—everything. The full catastrophe."*

Ah, yes. The "full catastrophe."

A curriculum on creating egalitarian relationships might include exercises on how to determine if each partner shares values and a common view of the future. *Children: yes or no? Bedroom window: open or closed? How important is it to "fight" fairly and forgive often?* But in the end, it is not those issues alone that make a relationship work for the long haul.

What might men in egalitarian relationships report? I suspect it would be very provocative but reassuring. To understand how best to create lives full of meaning, we must think deeply about how both people contribute to nurturing, sustained, and flexible loving partnerships.

Let me tell you about my Valentine . . .

My husband has received many "kudos" for playing nontraditional roles, yet when we both switched to four-day work weeks after the birth of our first child, colleagues were supportive of my choice but warned that it would "ruin his career." (Today, we are both tenured full professors.) When we share that he does most of the cooking, he gets showered with praise, yet my years of boiling the water for pasta or broiling the fish still go unacknowledged. Thus, as my experience exemplifies, egalitarian relationships are better for both partners but still require different sorts of internal and external negotiations for men. Attention to this, along with a reliable evidence base, could lead to greater flourishing for all of us.

Here comes my Valentine's Day theme. I have had the benefit of such an "egalitarian" loving partnership, and it has made all the difference. I met Mark in July 1984 when we were the interns on the 16 East medical team at Bellevue Hospital. Needless to say, we became very interdependent that summer, meeting regularly in the ICU to replace central lines or draw blood cultures, writing progress notes side-by-side well into the wee hours. I suspect there are few better ways to get to know a person's character than sharing a 2:00 am cup of cold "food truck" coffee. That summer, well before we became a couple, we were partners.

Mark recalls that time with much more "romance" than I do. He has always been the cornier one. I am the "realist," skeptical that romantic love even exists. I have been free with my feminist critique of all that life has thrown at us. He is the one who still believes in magic.

Over thirty-three years of marriage, there has been lots of tension and compromise. There were certainly many ways it could have—and almost did—go wrong. We have challenged assumptions, gained self-awareness, believed in and pushed each other, experimented, and occasionally jumped off the deep end. We never seem to get it exactly right, but we have gotten better at getting it close enough. We have made a home, raised children, and had our share of adventures. Our egalitarian relationship is a perpetual work in progress, more of a constant juggle than a harmonious balance. We are both better people because of it, and I might add, we have both found rewarding roles as clinician-scientists and administrators.

So, is this just good luck? Maybe. I certainly feel lucky. I know many of our junior colleagues think of us as a "dynamic duo." My response when I hear this is, "Forget the *Marvel Comics* version and come to dinner, see our messy but warm home, meet our kids and the cats, and watch us work it out."

On Joy and Sorrow in Our Long Winter

Ana Istrate, MD MS

In this essay published just days after the first vaccines became available, Dr. Istrate shared the emotional journey she experienced as a first-year internal medicine resident caring for desperately sick COVID-19 patients.

Then a woman said, Speak to us of Joy and Sorrow.
And he answered:
Your joy is your sorrow unmasked.
—Kahlil Gibran from "On Joy and Sorrow"

At the beginning of this strange year, I took a solo trip to Washington DC, a city I had never seen before. Sunlight hit the reflecting pool like a knife, the air was uncommonly warm, and the National Mall was full of maskless strangers. It was impossible to find a quiet moment at the Lincoln

Memorial. I met a family friend at the National Gallery of Art, where we made our way through currents of people, half in conversation with each other and half in conversation with the paintings and sculptures around us. I remember the contents of that conversation much less than I do the feeling of being in it, like floating on a raft through a luminous city, watching the threads of our childhood ripple in its wake.

It is curiously difficult to disentangle that more recent memory from all the memories of our lives that resurfaced then. Lately, I find myself running through the locales of my past as if turning the pages of a photo album, aware that I am looking for a particular photo without knowing exactly which one. There is no living memory that seems best poised to clarify our present trial.

Rotating through the COVID ICU

Fragments of time in the COVID ICU remain more salient than what took place there: squinting through the glass doors of negative pressure rooms to see if oxygen requirements had shifted or ventilator settings had been recalibrated, noticing the unforgiving brown-red of facial pressure ulcers as we prepared to place another line, and catching a glimpse of our medical student's eyes full of tears after our youngest patient had died. Equally vivid is the sensation of walking in each morning to be greeted by my co-residents' familiar faces. It went unstated, as many important things in our lives somehow do, but they fueled my optimism.

I remember placing the phone back in its cradle at the end of one of my night shifts, having told a wife—whose halting, soft voice I don't think I will ever forget—that her husband was not long for this world, only to find one of my co-residents sitting next to me, prepared with morning eyes to receive the story of that night. It's curious that we call these transitions of care "hand-offs." At times, it seems we redistribute emotional loads too.

Those of us who are interns have barely any point of reference for what being a physician was like before this pandemic, and we still spend much of our time taking care of non-COVID-19 patients. We take it on good faith that the medical ICU was busier and more strained this winter than the last. For better or for worse, this profession and its members stand firm in their resolve to soldier on. And so, the mental and emotional burden on all those involved in patient care is nothing new under the sun, but perhaps more profound.

I know I am not alone in the constant oscillation between hopefulness and seemingly impermeable disillusionment that this long season has brought us. There is a particular sting in the signs of indifference we encounter these days. It is present in the nonchalance of maskless strangers and the well-rehearsed backtracking of policymakers. Mercifully, we have little time to ruminate. That is the blessing of apprenticeship and its demands.

The thread unraveling behind us

And yet, that rushed, fragmented haste from one

patient or idea to the next bewilders us into forgetting that there is a thread unraveling behind us. Grief, rather than being reserved for clearly demarcated losses, is less a discrete emotion and more a slow change of climate. At its most acute, it leaves us in tears. But mostly, it is the inseparable string that links one loss to the next one in our lives. It becomes impossible to separate experiences, sleep deprivation notwithstanding. The death of my last patient in the ICU—a middle-aged, cadaverous man whose pancreatic disease marched him coldly into heart failure and whose death wish in his final hours left me heartbroken despite his ever-hostile (wounded) demeanor—had nothing to do with COVID-19, and yet I cannot extricate his story from the pandemic playing out in the background.

So many of us take comfort in relegating this year to the corner of exception. We are keen to label this pandemic an anomaly. It is with a perverse kind of thrill, too, that the media delights in labeling this moment (and the next) as a historical turning point. And there is no doubt that, given everything that has happened, it will be.

But how many of us can feel such cosmic shifts in our own inner worlds? It is frequently beyond the intimacy of human experience. Many of us have never confronted loss in such swift and raw a form, though we have been cognizant of it (I don't only mean the loss of life but also the loss of dignity and patience and faith). I wonder if we can forgive ourselves when it all seems so muddled and even collides with the small joys we still discover in our lives.

The view from here

Lately, there is more cause to hope than there has been in the past year, though I follow the news from the overwhelmed regions of the world with a heavy heart. A collective joy surrounds these early vaccination efforts, which stems from a deep sense of relief. I couldn't help but grin like a fool behind my mask as I felt the needle sink into my deltoid. (My vaccination card will be passed down through generations, I semi-jokingly tell my family and friends.)

The winter solstice is behind us, and a new year is about to begin. In six months of residency, I have encountered more kindness than I ever expected. The waters of the Reflecting Pool greet me every time my cell phone wakens, and the Lincoln Memorial sits in the corner of that photograph like an afterthought. Life has not yet given me cause to change the backdrop, though the thread has unraveled so fast and far from there. Somehow, there's no separating that afternoon from all the ones that followed.

Community Reflections: What is more noticeable in your life since our recent changes?

Wendy Peltier, MD, in Palliative Care, submitted this response:

"Sometimes your joy is the source of your smile, but sometimes, your smile can be the source of your joy."
—Thich Nhat Hanh

Spending so many of our days in masks has made me keenly aware of the power of a smile, and how challenging it is to not freely share expressions. Whether this might be with a fellow shopper or checkout assistant, a colleague at work, or when eagerly listening to a patient tell their story. Words seem strangely inadequate when not tied to sharing or reading facial expressions. The COVID-19 crisis has thrust us into times of fear and uncertainty, when this simple way to connect our humanity is strangely absent without a genuine replacement.

Community Reflections: What gives you a sense of peace at this time of year?

Jane Thelaner in Biophysics submitted this response:

A sunrise viewed from my office window, a crackling fire, twinkling candles, and holiday lights help me to defy the dark days of this long season. With the arrival of the winter solstice (technically the first day of winter), my faith in nature's rhythm evokes feelings of peace and hope that brighter days are ahead. Everything in its time . . .

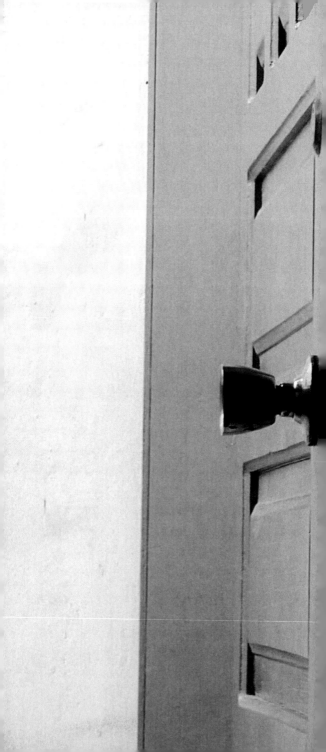

Spring 2021

The Messy

Cassie Ferguson, MD

*Dr. Ferguson, in this talk to the incoming Gold
Humanism Honor Society members, shared her
conviction that compassion for those who suffer must
be viewed through the lens of abundance rather than
scarcity. "Our capacity for compassion is endless."*

One very late night during my pediatric residency,
I sat in the middle of the pediatric intensive care unit
with my supervising fellow and the hospital chaplain.
A teenager we had been caring for had just chosen to
be decannulated (that is, have her tracheotomy tube
removed) and be allowed to die. She was sixteen years
old and had lived with a rare neuromuscular disease that
had progressed to the point that she could not breathe
without the aid of a ventilator and, more devastatingly,
could no longer paint or draw.

"Some days," the chaplain said, "some days, we are called to the messy."

Through the course of my career, I have been advised on how to wade through this mess—how to tend to the hardship, the pain, and the trauma experienced by the humans that we are called to care for and about. Well-meaning mentors have warned me to keep an emotional distance from my patients. Burnout experts warn us all of "compassion fatigue." Even the language we subconsciously revert to in the emergency department (ED) urges separation from human suffering—we care for "the broken arm in room 12" and "the non-accidental trauma in 5."

This perspective seems, to me, to arise from our deeply ingrained "culture of scarcity"; we can never have enough, know enough, be enough. We fear that our compassion is finite but that we just weren't told exactly when it would run out. So, we keep pushing and pushing, rightfully unwilling to ration it.

"Our capacity for compassion is endless"

I would like to offer a different perspective. I believe that our capacity for compassion is endless, that we can hold and attend to both the joy and the pain of our work, and that we can find meaning in and be transformed by the suffering we witness. For me, this begins with recognizing the limitations of empathy.

In a study using EEGs and MRIs, a team of social neuroscientists examined the differences between empathy and compassion. In one experiment, the French Buddhist monk, Matteau Ricard, was asked to listen to recorded sounds of a woman screaming with the specific instruction to feel her distress but do nothing more. The pain centers of his brain were active, and he struggled to continue. Then he was instructed to listen to the same sounds, but to also engage in compassion meditation — to repeat phrases offering up safety, health, and ease to this person. His pain centers remained activated but so, too, were the neural networks associated with love and other positive emotions. He felt that he could continue to do this indefinitely.

Empathy is affective resonance with someone else; it allows you to feel suffering when they suffer and to feel joy when they feel joy. Empathic resonance alone, however, can lead to emotional distress and burnout. "Empathy," Ricard writes, "should take place within the much vaster space" of compassion and love.

It is important to unpack this term with the intention of understanding what it is, how it serves our patients, and how we cultivate it. Ricard wrote beautifully that "compassion is nothing else than love applied to suffering." Empathy directs our attention to where it hurts; compassion calls us to work to understand the levels of pain, and the manifest and latent causes of it, so that we might effectively help and empower. Compassion calls us to act, to engage with our patients and with our communities.

Cultivating this compassion and sustaining it through the demands of our profession is effortful; caring for self while caring for others should be a daily practice held with the same reverence that you hold doctoring. That practice will look differently for each of you. But I urge you to keep these key components in mind:

- First, pause frequently. Intentionally make space for rest, recovery, and being still. For me, this has looked like asking our team to pause together after a death in the ED and taking back some of the hours lost to my smartphone to be in solitude.

- Second, stay fully present in your experience no matter how difficult. This is as straightforward as stopping to notice and name the emotions coming up for you during patient encounters. After sitting with a mom who just learned her five-year-old has leukemia, it is easy to do what Brené Brown calls "overfunction"; rather than recognize how our emotions are impacting us, we jump to reassure, and to fix, and to plan. If I sit and say to myself, "I am feeling fear," or "I am feeling anger," I can remain present for her and let compassion guide my actions instead.

- And lastly, as the meditation teacher Jack Kornfield wrote, "If your compassion does not include yourself, it is incomplete."

Compassion in practice

A few weeks ago, I sat with a student during their dismissal hearing. The experience was understandably distressing for them, and I struggled to help. So, I consciously engaged in a practice that I use nearly every shift in the ED, one that some of you have heard me talk about before; I sat across from them and noticed my breathing. With every inhale I thought about breathing in compassion for myself, and with every exhale I breathed out compassion for them. I know that even this small departure from focusing on others makes some of us uncomfortable and makes us feel as if we are abandoning our mission as caretakers. But in that moment, with that student, rather than feeling overwhelmed and reflexively pulling away or trying to fix, I felt only love. And love, far from sentimentality, is the force that undergirds the most important and transformative moments in humankind's history.

Love is also the way through; we must harness it if we are to continue to alleviate the suffering of others, fight for social justice, and care for our communities and our planet in a sustainable and intentional way. As I have learned often during my career, patients, caregivers, and the world around us are all wading through "the messy." They each deserve my best efforts to provide them with my mindful attention, my love, and my compassion.

Providing Space to Shed Tears May Be Key to a Better, Post-COVID Future

Adina Kalet, MD MPH

As the shutdowns wore on, Dr. Kalet shared data that demonstrates the disproportionate effect of the pandemic on women, both at MCW and nationally.

Over the past couple of weeks, I have witnessed more tears among my colleagues and mentees than I normally see in a year. Even though I care deeply, I am not particularly worried about those who have cried. I find it reassuring that they reached out, seeking support and a reliable pep talk. I know that while shedding tears in someone else's presence makes one vulnerable, it is also a sign of strength, resilience, and self-care. These individuals are bending under the prolonged pressures of the COVID-19 pandemic but are unlikely to break.

On January 21, 2021, Libby Ellinas, MD, Director

of the MCW Center for the Advancement of Women in Science and Medicine (AWSM), Associate Dean for Women's Leadership, and Professor of Anesthesiology at MCW, gave Kern Institute Grand Rounds on Women in COVID-19. Her talk was a tour de force of cautionary tales and sobering data. She reminded us that the majority of people on the front lines of healthcare and education—and nearly half of our medical school faculty—are women. Data from multiple sources are consistent: women as a group are under special pressures during this pandemic. This poses a threat to both our medical education and healthcare systems.

The ways in which COVID-19 has disproportionately affected women

Dr. Ellinas shared survey data from the USC Dornsife Center for Economic and Social Research confirming that the mental load—including concerns about the health of their families, themselves, and financial strain—is significantly higher among women compared with men. And while married men with children have the lowest mental distress, women with children have, by far, the highest. This is not news. Sociologists have shown over-and-over that being married with children is associated with better health and more happiness for men while, for women, being married/partnered with children is associated with relatively high levels of stress and distress. Women do measurably more emotional work than men, both in families and at work. While often this work is energizing, it is a mental load that can overwhelm.

Among MCW faculty members, Dr. Ellinas demonstrated that the social isolation necessitated by the pandemic is wreaking havoc for working women. With schools inconsistently in session, direct childcare hours have increased for both men and women, but the number of additional hours per week has been greater for women. Data from an MCW AWSM COVID-19 survey shows that while nearly 60% of male faculty have spouses employed part-time or not at all, this is true for only 21% of female faculty. Thus, MCW working women with families are much less likely to have robust support systems than their male counterparts.

There is also heterogeneity in how COVID-19 increases stress. Some find value in working from home, but many do not. Clearly, working from home—for those privileged to be able to do so—allows more flexibility and autonomy, reduces time spent commuting, and decreases costs associated with working away from home. It might even provide unexpected "quality time" with family. However, especially for working women with school-aged children, working from home is associated with less sleep and decreased self-care. Adding to this, the intersectionality of race and gender can weigh even more heavily on Black and Brown women.

And, as if that wasn't challenging enough, there are signs that the COVID-19 pandemic negatively impacts the academic productivity of early-career women more than it does men. The long-term impact of this is worrisome and may lead to the reversal of recent gains in women's academic status on the whole. These are challenges for us all.

Institutional solutions are critical and complex

What did Dr. Ellinas recommend? She offered a number of institutional recommendations that are consistent with AWSM's inspiring and audacious vision that *"MCW will be a destination for women leaders, cultivating an inclusive and vibrant culture that supports all genders to grow and thrive in the health sciences,"* and mission *"to advance the careers of women at MCW through data-informed strategic projects that enhance opportunity and improve workplace climate."*

- Evaluating leadership structures to ensure women are well represented in decision-making
- Valuing parenting through generous parental leave and creative childcare
- Supporting women to "step forward" rather than depending on "step back" policies
- Valuing the hard work of mentoring, equity, diversity, and inclusion
- Valorizing women role models for us all

We need policies that can be individualized and flexible over time. Extraordinary caregiving responsibilities may be *acute*, due to an illness or urgent need; *chronic*, as in having a child with special needs or an aging relative with evolving needs; or *both*, as in this stuttering pandemic. Community resources are distributed unevenly. Some people do not have enough help while others have what they need, if not to excess. Institutions like ours can improve the quality of life for our employees and community by offering concrete services, such as low-cost, high-quality childcare, sick childcare, food preparation and delivery, and help with chores.

To support women (and men) whose academic careers have been impacted by the pandemic, some institutions have found ways to provide assistance that enable researchers to continue collecting and analyzing data while they tend to a "special" personal need. One program, the Doris Duke Fund for the Retention of Clinical Scientists, has funded such efforts. Many workplaces provide access to high quality food, recreation, and other wellness services. Much can be done.

How do we, as an institution, come out of COVID-19 better and stronger? We need a flexible range of options going forward that includes working from home. Our men need to engage. We all need to honestly complete surveys to have quality data that informs best solutions. Men who have the relative privilege of having more support at home and at work—as well as having disproportionately higher salaries—need to be allies and advocates for equity and flexibility. No one should assume that they, alone, know what will work; we need to ask women. Don't insist on "fairness" or "equality" until you have a full-thickness view of the situation.

Back to crying

I have always kept a box of tissues on my desk. When seeing patients, the box was discreetly tucked just out of view, easily slid toward the patient at the first glisten in the eyes. As a colleague and mentor, the box would be brought forward when the face flushed, the head dropped, and the tears rolled. It has been my experience that, most of the time, a good cry in the presence of an empathic other is the most efficient way to clear the air and help the words and problem-solving flow. People cry for all sorts of reasons. Sometimes it is sadness and grief, but just as often people cry because they are overwhelmed, angry, or frustrated. I have come to believe that an effective mentor, like the good physician, must learn to invite and sit with the tears of others without needing to fix anything; just listen, sit quietly, check in. Fighting back tears takes energy, blocks thinking, and keeps others away. Letting tears fall clears the air and loosens the voice.

Did I say that it is mostly women who shed tears in my office? Well, it is. But occasionally, the men cry as well. Three times in the past three weeks, I have spoken with distraught educational leaders, people who are deeply respected by colleagues and beloved by trainees. They were emotionally and physically exhausted from the expanding and rapidly evolving needs of school-aged children and elderly parents. They had less help from their working spouse than they needed. Their jobs presented new and growing demands on themselves and their trainees (e.g., being "deployed" to care for critically ill COVID-19 patients). They feared a loss of income. They were at the brink.

In each case, I pushed the virtual box of tissues. *Why doesn't Zoom design a "tissue box" emoji?* I hope my message is clear: It is okay to cry here. I am not afraid of your tears. I will hear you out and empathize. You are not crazy, this is hard. I know you will find your way through this. I will help if I can.

These folks do not need to be fixed, they just need a shoulder to cry on, a good night's rest, regular meals, and an occasional walk in the woods. I think we can get them that.

I Am Not Your Model Minority

Maya Saravanan

MCW student Maya Saravanan shared instances of microaggressions and stereotype threat that she has experienced during her journey to medical school.

I stood at her desk to ask for a hall pass so that I could use the restroom. She looked down at the roster.

"Hmm . . . This name here, Vishmayaa Saravanan? Is that you?"

I glanced around the room at my white classmates, then back at her. I appreciated her for not jumping to conclusions, but she had to admit that was a good one.

"Yep."

"You're Indian? My neighbor's Indian."

Congratulations. And no, I don't know them.

"Yes, I am."

"So, are you going to be a doctor, engineer, or

something like that, right? My neighbor's a doctor. I read there are special visas for Indians to come over and work in those fields—pretty neat stuff. Model minority. We need more smart people like you."

Later that night, my thoughts raced...As a high school senior, I was starting to explore the idea of one day becoming a physician. Yet, I couldn't help but wonder how much of my dream was influenced by cultural stereotypes and expectations placed upon me from an incredibly young age. My parents and I immigrated from Chennai, India, where I was born. As my substitute teacher so aptly suggested, my father was able to arrive on an H1B visa for labor. He and my mother were amongst the few to leave the villages they once called home. To leave that environment and come to Pittsburgh, Pennsylvania provided about as drastic of a culture shock as existed. Despite their basic education and unawareness of the US schooling system, they stayed determined to put their children through school. Thus, it's no surprise that for my entire childhood, I was hyper-aware of the sacrifices my parents had made to prioritize my brother and me. To this day, I'm unsure of how I could ever begin to repay them for building us a life here from the ground up. Yet, this narrative isn't specific to me—many first-generation immigrants feel an undue burden of having to perform at the highest level, for fear that anything less will invalidate their family's entire journey.

After college, I completed a year-long fellowship in the nonprofit sector to develop my leadership skills. We met with many impactful Pittsburgh leaders. Corroborating my previous experiences, I noticed that very few of them looked like me. My identity as a South Asian, oldest daughter of humble immigrants, and doctor-to-be was almost wholly defined as being the stereotypical model minority. If this, in fact, the "American dream," why weren't there more of us in leadership? Why did our examples of strong leaders continue to be those who don't share my perspective? Why was I shamed for looking vastly different from the guy next door, but was still expected to outperform him ten times over?

These weren't the only existential questions I faced. As a woman, I struggle to find the balance between "aggressive" and "confident." Having darker skin, I wonder if I would be considered more beautiful if my skin was lighter. As a first-generation student, I play medical medium at my parents' doctor appointments, interpreting terms like "sagittal and coronal planes" while only just having learned them myself. Stumbling through these doubts, I see the term "model minority" and find that I would describe myself as anything but. However difficult to navigate, the intersectionality of my core—combined with the nuances of each identity—have been well received in my new endeavors in leadership. Institutionally, and across our nation, there are endless arenas in which mass cultural change must be immediate. I've been privileged with multiple opportunities to showcase my leadership in a way that doesn't stifle my identity but rather celebrates it, and allows me to speak and act confidently to create change.

I believe everyone's experiences directly shape their leadership style and, thus, their interactions with others. In working with leaders who have trouble relating to my shared experience, my past leadership style was defined by accepting complacency and hesitating to speak up for fear of being dismissed. The more I work with leaders who provide a safe environment, the more I feel comfortable speaking up against policies that reinforce generational trauma and racism, and speaking less when others need a platform. With the support of administrators, professors, and fellow students, I'm learning that mistakes are inevitable and part of the journey to betterment. Finally, through self reflection, I'm accepting that the toxic model minority myth suppresses members of our community from using their experiences to lead in an individualistic and honest way. Yes, our race shapes us, but it is not a way to infer what we are capable of. I am entering medicine because I believe that quality in communal mental and physical health is a crucial component to the success of the public, not because it's what Indians come to the United States for.

While I have a long way to go in developing each of my identities through leadership, I'm thankful to be working through my experiences and finding value in what once held me back. I will always lean on my upbringing to give back to the country that welcomed my family and me twenty-five years ago. At my core, I am a South Asian woman, a daughter of immigrants, and an almost-physician. But I am not your model minority. An homage to my substitute teacher— pretty neat stuff indeed.

Teaching is Love

Megan Schultz, MD MA

Dr. Schultz, who taught Spanish in an urban Baltimore high school before going into medicine, shared the story of the student who inspired her to become a doctor.

Before I was a doctor, I was a teacher. I taught Spanish at Frederick Douglass High School in Baltimore for two years before I decided to go to medical school. It was one of my students, Torreantoe Smalls, who inspired me to become a doctor. Torry was mischievous, with a quick grin. He played the trumpet like nobody's business and tried, sweetly and patiently, to teach my clueless, clumsy feet how to step dance. He once got a B+ on a Spanish exam, and even though he was just beside himself with pride, he made me swear up and down I wouldn't tell anyone he had actually studied for it. During his senior year, Torry was shot multiple times in the abdomen during an attempted robbery. He would ultimately spend two years and three months of his life in the hospital, enduring dozens of surgeries and losing nearly two feet of bowel. It was in his hospital room, staring at his small frame in the bed, surrounded by the clicks and beeps of machines, that I resolved to become a doctor.

Fifteen years later, here I am: a doctor, yes, but also still a teacher. Instead of high school students, now I teach medical students, residents, and fellows. Instead of teaching people how to speak Spanish, now I teach people how to be doctors. This is a tall order; sometimes it's hard to know what to prioritize. When I was in medical school myself, I often felt impatient and restless, like none of my professors really understood the point of being a doctor at all. They talked way too much about things like the Henderson-Hasselbach equation and not nearly enough about how to save the life of someone like Torry. And the way they taught! PowerPoint slide after PowerPoint slide, crammed with text in a tiny font that I was expected to regurgitate on command. I have often thought that medical school would be far more interesting and effective if it were taught by good teachers who know nothing about medicine as opposed to good doctors who know nothing about teaching. But how to be a good teacher for medical trainees? How to balance the need for basic physiologic knowledge with broad themes of compassion and empathy? I decided to ask the person who inspired me to be a doctor in the first place: I decided to call Torry.

Torry is not Torry anymore; he is Mr. Smalls. He is now a teacher himself; he teaches percussion at Mervo

High School in Baltimore. He is also father to three children and runs an entertainment company called TORKO ENT. He still has the mischievous grin—but the speed at which it appears has been tempered a bit by age and wisdom. I asked Torry what makes a good teacher. His answer was arrestingly simple: love.

Torry described the importance of love by telling me the story of Mr. B., his music teacher at Douglass High. Torry had met Mr. B. when he auditioned for the Douglass Marching Band as a skinny eighth grader—and from the beginning, Mr. B. believed in him and acted like a father figure to him. "He was the first person to see who I really was," Torry says. After he was shot, Mr. B. regularly visited Torry in the hospital. One of the days Mr. B. was visiting, he was asked to step out so the nurses could give Torry a bath. For months, Torry could not move his legs, stand, or walk. As a result, he had to rely on nurses for sponge baths in bed, which he described as a singularly humiliating experience. "You know, I'm cool, so I don't want nobody giving me a sponge bath. But I didn't have no choice!" he said with that old grin.

Torry said, "This was when I knew Mr. B. loved me as a son . . . After my [bath], after my visitors came back in, I was sitting there in bed trying to lotion myself. And I was so mad that I couldn't move my legs, that I couldn't reach my feet. The man took the lotion—I didn't even ask him—he just saw me struggling." And Mr. B. knew what to do. The memory of Mr. B. empathizing with him in that moment, selflessly helping Torry with such a basic need, still moved Torry to tears fifteen years later. "He made me feel that I was loved," Torry said.

To love our students—it's not often something we talk about as teachers. But maybe it is love that's the foundation of any successful student-teacher connection: to believe in our students, to know what to do when they are struggling, to help them without being asked. Maybe if we start from a place of compassion and empathy, all the basic physiologic knowledge will follow.

Without Torry, I don't know if I would be a doctor today. I certainly wouldn't be the same type of doctor. All my students in Baltimore taught me far more than I ever taught them—Torry is the perfect example of that. There is such beauty in knowing that he is a teacher now, seeing his students for who they really are, believing in them, loving them. Torreantoe Smalls: once my student, always my teacher.

Seeking Wisdom in COVID-19 Times

Adina Kalet, MD MPH

In this essay, published one year after COVID-19 first shut down the US, Dr. Kalet mused on the capacities needed to generate wisdom from our shared experiences of the pandemic and its aftermath.

We are weary. The COVID-19 pandemic drags on and, while spring is in the air and an end to our social isolation seems in sight, many of us feel traumatized. I do not need to review our losses except to say there have been many—we will be feeling them for a while—and some people will be marked for life. There will be long-term negative consequences. We can only hope there might also be growth.

Philosophers and psychologists agree that the human capacity to find steadiness or growth in the face of challenge is often the path to wisdom, or as a colleague of mine used to regularly opine during our nights on call, *"just another f--king growth experience."*

In the first six months of the pandemic, Tyler VanderWeele, PhD, epidemiologist, biostatistician, and director of the Human Flourishing Program at Harvard University, studied a national sample of adults. Remarkably, he demonstrated that the domains of *Meaning and Purpose and Character and Virtue* held steady in the face of this adversity! Not surprisingly, other domains, including *Happiness and Life Satisfaction, Mental and Physical Health, Close Social Relationships, and Financial and Material Stability*, declined. It tells us that, while we have all been traumatized over the past year and have experienced the impact, most of us are still capable of "post-traumatic growth."

Wisdom practices: "What COVID-19 has taught me"

I have a friend who keeps a running list of *"What COVID-19 has taught me."* The list reminds her daily of her post-traumatic growth and, although much of it is tongue-in-cheek (e.g., fourth grade math, what a spike protein is), the list continues to expand. Establishing habits centered around gratitude is a characteristic of a wise person.

This past week, I (virtually) attended a conference sponsored by the Wake Forest University Program for Leadership and Character and cosponsored by the Oxford Character Project entitled "Character and the Professions." Thought-leaders from religion, business, engineering and technology, public life, law and, of course, medicine gave talks and engaged in panel discussions around the "crisis of character in leadership." In olden pre-pandemic times, all the attendees would have traveled to Winston-Salem, North Carolina, checked into hotels, hobnobbed with each other wearing plastic badges on lanyards, sat together in large auditoriums, and watched the inspiring speakers (Colin Powell and Madeleine Albright!) on jumbotrons. Instead, the 2,300 participants "Zoomed" in from the comfort of their own homes in thirty-seven countries, sat in their own time zones and, probably, participated in pajamas; I did dress up and put on lipstick—but no high heels—for the one session where I was on camera, just for old time's sake.

The conference experience reminded me that there have been so many losses in this virtual world. We cannot catch up with old friends and make unanticipated, new connections. We miss the chance to travel, experience new cultures, and have long conversations over shared meals.

Yet, the trade-offs are worth celebrating. As was the Kern Institute's experience with our large events this past year, this past week's conference touched a much larger, more geographically diverse audience and, of course, everyone saved a tremendous amount of time, money, and jet fuel. We still had meaningful conversations about important ideas. This is on my *"What COVID-19 has taught me"* gratitude list. I learned a great deal.

Practical Wisdom and Virtuous Cycles: How do we help learners turn obstacles into growth?

At the Kern Institute, we propose that attaining Practical Wisdom is a central goal of medical education. Practical Wisdom, or *phronesis* in Greek, is the ability to *"do the right thing, at the right time, for the right reasons."* Sounds good, right? But how exactly do we educate toward wisdom?

In her talk at the conference, Margaret Plews-Ogan, MD (Chief of the Division of General Medicine, Geriatrics, and Palliative Medicine at University of Virginia School of Medicine) pointed out that *"we are in most need of wisdom when things are most uncertain and ambiguous."* As any physician recognizes, the daily practice of our profession provides endless wisdom learning opportunities.

But what is wisdom, really? (You might want to read this paragraph twice . . .) It has been conceptualized as "a set of reflective, cognitive, and affective capacities which can be learned and honed—usually most effectively through facing adversity—and engaging in a particular kind of reflection intentionally aimed at meaning-making and increasing tolerance for uncertainty and ambiguity, compassion, and humility."

What is key here? It is that this reflection goes beyond understanding and managing one's own emotional states, because a wise person focuses on the greater good, not simply one's own.

If we longitudinally integrate opportunities for such reflection in our education, we turn challenges into opportunities to promote both individual well-being and wisdom. To be a "virtuous cycle" that leads to growth rather than despair, obstacles must be linked with a teacher-guided acceptance, reflection, meaning-making, and integration in order to create a new sense of self or identity formation. The cycle strengthens the character of individuals and transforms our learning contexts and environments into places where we can explicitly and intentionally foster wisdom.

Opportunities and challenges to the development of Practical Wisdom

COVID-19 aside (a big aside!), medical training and practice provide opportunities for— but do not guarantee—the development of Practical Wisdom. There is the possibility of both <u>Post-Traumatic Growth</u> (the positive impacts gained by struggling with highly stressful, traumatic life events) alongside <u>Post-Traumatic Stress</u> (those noxious, persistent, and disturbing psychological impacts of trauma). There is the possibility of the trainee entering a <u>Virtuous Cycle </u>(where each obstacle provides a growth opportunity) or a <u>Vicious Cycle</u> (that carries the trainee further and further down).

As educators, how do we live and model this? We must practice being open to traumatic experiences and incline ourselves towards gratitude and forgiveness. These traits will predispose us to experience wisdom formation in the midst of trauma. Will we include more compassion and connectedness as we discover new paths? Will we develop a greater appreciation for life and ask deeper philosophical questions?

As educators, we must ensure that our trainees experience growth even as they have experienced disquiet. Attentive mentors working within cultures of character and caring can be changemakers. As we approach the light at the end of the pandemic tunnel, let's seek to be wiser for our patients, our students, our families, and ourselves.

Interviewing for Fellowships— My 2020 Experience

David A Campbell, MD

Dr. Campbell, who was completing his residency at the time, wrote about the uncharted waters of interviewing for fellowships virtually.

"Please tell me you're not in Atlanta yet!"

It was March 12, 2020, the day before my first fellowship interview. In the days preceding, interviews dropped off the calendar one by one as travel restrictions tightened and hospital campuses closed their doors to nonessential workers. Some programs switched directly to virtual interviews, while others were hopeful they could have applicants in person by May or June (a wildly optimistic prospect, in hindsight). The Atlanta program finally shut their campus down, and the coordinator was frantically trying to stop applicants from getting on flights.

After getting through medical school and residency interviews, I knew this would be very different. However, as I worked through nineteen virtual interviews spanning five months, I did find some surprises along the way.

The first thought was how disappointing it was to be unable to visit the cities and hospitals I'd potentially be spending a year at. A very close second thought (in reality, probably a simultaneous thought) was how much money I'd save. Already, credit card bills were piling up and vacation days were evaporating. It was becoming clear that physically getting to nineteen interviews was likely going to be impossible. However, on the virtual interview trail, I could attend a morning interview in Florida, an afternoon interview in California, and an evening Zoom social event in New York, all without leaving my apartment or spending a dime. Some programs scattered interviews over several days, meaning I could duck into a hospital workroom for fifteen minutes at a time, using no vacation days at all. I'll admit I did several interviews between cases wearing a suit coat and scrub pants.

Some aspects of the virtual process weren't immediately obvious. One significant drawback was not meeting the other applicants. Otolaryngology is a small enough specialty that during the residency interview trail, applicants tend to run into each other several times. In the process of comparing notes on past and future interviews at social events or making small talk on the tenth hospital tour, many of us formed connections that only grew as we found each other at conferences throughout residency and will continue to grow as we move through our careers. The graduating ENT class of 2021 got to meet each other during the interview trail of 2016. Now, as I was virtually interviewing to enter the even smaller community of Head and Neck Surgical Oncology, I realized I was missing out on the opportunity to meet my soon-to-be colleagues.

There were also some unexpected advantages to virtual interviews. As interviews approached, there was concern if programs and applicants could get to know each other as well on the virtual platforms. Similar to the residency match, the ten-to-fifteen-minute interviews themselves are incredibly important for both applicant and program. A single awkward interaction vs. a meaningful connection can have huge impacts on how applicants and programs rank each other. Of course, there were the expected technological hiccups with lots of *"I can hear you. Can you hear me?"* However, I had several interviews that felt easier because they were virtual.

While many physicians interviewed from their offices, I spoke to several world-famous Head and Neck surgeons from their homes. One particularly well-known surgeon was arriving home from work as the interview started. He greeted and introduced me to his wife and showed off the view from his yard (*"This could be the type of view you get if you move here!"*). From the applicant's side, rather than being led into an office at an unfamiliar hospital after sleeping in a hotel bed, I was often interviewing from my apartment with my cats napping on my bed that was just steps away. While some ability to connect was undoubtedly lost with interviews being virtual, my guess is that both parties being in a familiar setting facilitated easier connections in a different way that would not have been possible in-person.

I've heard the sentiment over and over that virtual interviews could never replace in-person interviews. In many ways, I agree with this. However, it was refreshing to see people finding new ways to connect with each other when the world was turned upside down.

Work and Career in that Order: Residency is Just the Next Step in the Life of a Physician

Adina Kalet, MD MPH

On Residency Match Day 2021, Dr. Kalet published this essay celebrating the creativity of the first medical school class to move on to residencies without the benefit of in-person interviews or away rotations. She offers the newly matched students some advice, because how they view their residency training will shape the kinds of physicians they will become.

Later today, more than 48,000 medical students will find out where they will begin residency training in July.

While the numbers vary, about half of students matched to their top choice, and about two-thirds to one of their top three. About 5% of all applicants did not match and have spent the week working with deans and faculty to "scramble" into open slots. There will be disappointments, and not everyone will be thrilled.

In normal times, MCW-Milwaukee would be hosting our 200 students, their families, and their friends in an Alumni Center celebration with balloons, short speeches, finger food, intense excitement, and identical "I MATCHED!!!" t-shirts. Even still, today's celebration and energy will be shared on social media and over the internet when, at noon EDT, students open the e-equivalent of an "envelope" and learn for the first time to which program they have matched.

Today is one of the most significant watershed moments in each of their lives. They will, finally, be able to glimpse more clearly the outlines of their future selves.

The importance of "place" in residency training

Where a physician trains does matter. Residency takes each young physician to a city or town where they are committed to stay for a while and, although it varies by specialty, over 50% of physicians end up practicing in the state where they complete training. The shared experience of residency builds profound and lifelong friendships forged during long nights on-call and the intellectual, physical, and emotional challenges inherent with the transition from medical student to practicing physician. Clinical "habits" are formed and imprinted for a lifetime.

I am amazed how intense the experiences I had during my own residency remain. While I have not drawn blood cultures, done a lumbar puncture, or placed central intravenous line in the subclavian vein in three decades, I still recall the rhythm of each procedure, the proper aseptic techniques, the positioning of the patient, the feel of the cannulas and needles, and the proper documentation. My fingers remember the sensation of the needle overcoming resistance, piercing the skin, and finding the proper space. During my residency, I learned to rehearse "delivering bad news," and still do so as I walk toward a difficult conversation. Facing an emergency, I still summon courage the same way I did when I was wearing the "code beeper" and running toward, rather than away from, the crisis. *Always take the stairs. Never wait for the elevator. Hope the nurses are already there with the cart. Will the medical student by my side be ready to do chest compressions?* I learned to be ready when I arrived.

Looking for meaning during residency training

Some things have changed about the match since I was in medical school. While many of my classmates in the early 1980s applied to only one type of residency, a sizable minority listed more than one type of program on their match lists, allowing the algorithm to determine whether they would end up as an internist, pediatrician, dermatologist, or orthopedist. I share this because I now know how this approach worked out. These peripatetic students understood something the rest of us did not, and here is the lesson: It is much more important to choose *what kind of career* you want to have, than *which clinical discipline or "tribe"* you seek to join. They understood that there are, for most of us, many paths to a satisfying life as a physician.

Here are some examples. One friend knew she wanted to spend her career in women's health, so she applied to and ranked OB/Gyn, family medicine, and internal medicine programs. Another close colleague, hoping for a quiet, suburban, "Marcus Welby" type of practice, applied to both family medicine and internal medicine. They let the match decide their specialty, knowing that each path would lead to their goals. Other classmates were so committed to *where* they wanted to live that they applied to several different specialties in the same city, believing that the type of residency was secondary.

This type of flexibility seems very old-fashioned now, and there are reasons for this. Over the past decades, for example, the increase in medical school graduates has far outpaced the increase in first-year residency positions, placing an intense *"What if I don't match?"* pressure on students that we never experienced. Today, certain clinical fields are so competitive that students feel the need to plan far ahead, take time off to complete specialty-focused research, concentrate on doing things that will make them more attractive for the few spots, and audition extensively. Back when each residency program had its own pen-and-paper application form, we applied to ten or so institutions and ranked five to eight. These days, the number of electronic applications submitted by each applicant continues to climb, and it is not unusual for a medical student to apply to over sixty programs hoping for a handful of interviews. Different times, for sure. But instructive. Life as a physician has always been a journey with many choices, and residency is just the next step after medical school.

"Careers are made in retrospect."

Most of us can look back and see the paths we took, the opportunities we seized, and the roads not taken. But discerning the path that still lies ahead of us is impossible. It is rare to meet someone who, in retrospect, knew where they were going from the very beginning. Nearly half of the students who match today are entering different fields than they had envisioned for themselves when they started medical school. As many as 20% of residents switch fields before the end of their training. Mid-career physicians often retrain into new clinical specialties, seek advanced education, or pursue mid-career fellowships in a wide range of areas.

My women's health friend, for example, ended up happily doing groundbreaking immigrant health research. "Marcus Welby" is now a professor and urban health services researcher. Even though they did not end up where they might have predicted, their training gave them the flexibility to build satisfying and meaningful careers.

This is really good news. It means we can each feel free to be fully in the present. With reflection, mentorship, and opportunity, we can redirect our work. As the ancient Greeks advised: Know thyself. Then move in that direction.

The wonder of a career in medicine is its flexibility and ever-emerging opportunities. So how do we make good choices?

Residency is a learning experience, but it is also a job. Some advice . . .

Find work that matters. Look for the aspects of your new careers that intrigue you and get you out of bed in the morning. As novice physicians, you will learn about yourselves and your patients as you engage with both the well and the chronically ill. You will learn to prioritize and lead teams as you work through the daily tasks and confront the patients who decompensate in front of you. You will perform procedures that require significant manual dexterity and employ advanced technology. You will engage with colleagues, team members, and communities. You will collect and analyze data, peer through microscopes, study the results of sophisticated analyzers, and seek the truth and beauty hidden in a radiologic image. You will deal with unimaginable ambiguity. Learn to think, to feel, and to engage at various paces and rhythms — optimally, for your entire professional lifetime.

Take time to reflect and grow. Listen to others as they help you discern how your work impacts you. Find ways to stay well even as you do the hardest work in your life.

Residency is only one step on the path to a career

Training is extremely hard, and it can become a life of one challenge after another. Yet, as residents touch the lives of patients, learners, colleagues, friends, family, and the community, opportunities for growth, character development, and change-making present themselves. Some residents will avoid these occasions while others will seek them out. To some, the work of residency will drive them forward into rich careers, dictating their goals and what they work on. For others, the opportunities will fade into the background while they are "busy making other plans."

This is what continues to astonish me. While residency is an overwhelming experience, there are those who take full advantage of its opportunities. They learn early that training is only one step toward a career that will take unexpected twists along the way. As faculty, we must recognize their sacrifices, yet help them stop and consider: *What do you want to be able to say you have done? How will you know you have done it, influenced others, engaged in those conversations, made the world just a little better? How might I help?*

And there have been upsides!

Programs saw the numbers of applicants increase. There was a more diverse applicant pool. Web pages were spiffy, social media campaigns were buffed, and all hands were on deck as residents showcased their program's camaraderie and the wonders of living in Milwaukee. In some ways more exhausting (Zoom fatigue) and in some ways more intimate, faculty and applicants got to see each other's home offices and meet the family dog. No cheese curds, brats, and beer; instead, there were suit jackets, a clean shave, and a new house plant along with scrub pants and sneakers.

Creativity overflows. This is an important moment. Let's take advantage of it.

How to Plan a Pandemic Wedding

Sophia Kiernan

Ms. Kiernan, an MCW-Milwaukee medical student, had more than merely classwork on her mind as the pandemic closed in. In this essay, she shared her story of changing her wedding plans with lots of help from family and friends.

———————————

Step 1: Book your wedding venue sixteen months in advance. You know you want to get married in Green Bay, and you know pickings are slim in the Green Bay wedding venue market. Filter by ones that will hold your and your fiancé's massive families. Then filter by ones that serve something other than broasted chicken—if you're not sure if they serve something other than broasted chicken, call the owners. Most will be shocked that you want something other than broasted chicken.

Step 2: Book a rehearsal dinner venue, specifically the venue you have been planning to have your rehearsal dinner in since you were twelve (the only part of your wedding you've had planned since you were twelve).

Step 3: Marvel at how on top of the game you are, and don't worry much about wedding planning for many months. Wedding planning? It's not that hard, right?

Step 4: Receive email from rehearsal dinner venue that they are closing their restaurant that has been a staple in Green Bay for decades. Darn. Can you believe that? Our rehearsal venue closed! How unlucky are we? Oh well, it's just the rehearsal dinner!

Step 5: Enter stage left—global pandemic. It's February! We're getting married in June! This will all be fine by then.

Step 6: It's not fine.

Step 7: Figure out "disaster backup plan" that involves one-sixth of your guest list.

Step 8: Coordinate Wedding 1.0 for 2020 while simultaneously coordinating Wedding 2.0 for 2021 with the original venue.

Step 9: Set plan in motion and marvel at how flexible you are. Make a cute video with your fiancé announcing the news. Make sure everyone knows that you're handling it like a champ, and that it's all going to be okay. You're coordinating two weddings and are practically 25% a doctor. You're unstoppable.

Step 10: Receive call that the original venue is closing, effective immediately, and you are now competing with 100 couples for those previously mentioned broasted chicken venues.

Return to Step 1.

The good news? We did get married on our originally

planned wedding date of June 13, 2020. It was certainly not the wedding we had spent a year and a half planning; a 300-person guest list and COVID-19 weren't exactly compatible. My husband, Nathan, and I have always identified as being "big wedding people" and we both come from big families with lots of cousins we love. A small wedding wasn't even on the table when we started planning. In March 2020, we started writing a "disaster plan" of what we would do if we could only have fifty people, but we didn't seriously think we'd have to actually uninvite 250 people from our wedding. As it got closer and closer, however, we realized that we were going to have to become small wedding people, and fast.

I read a book early on in the wedding planning process about "practical" planning. It said to let other people help you; you have so many people in your life who love you, and those people have skills. Let them use those skills to help you pull off a wedding. While I thought this was a lovely idea, I felt like this was supposed to be a party that we planned and other people enjoyed. My guests aren't supposed to be having to help me make sure they enjoy it by tying ribbons on pews or baking desserts. *And then* God probably just laughed at me. Because the only way you can replan a wedding in one month during a global pandemic is to get a ton of help from people who love you.

We had a crowdsourced wedding, through and through. My godparents immediately offered their gorgeous backyard as a reception venue. My brothers played five instruments between the three of them at our Mass. Our friends sanitized the entire church while we took pictures. My aunt offered to make cheesecake for fifty people. Basically, our guests were the only reason we successfully pulled off this wedding, and that made our wedding even more wonderful.

It's easy to think of a wedding as being about two people. And it is, in many ways, because I was the one in the white dress and Nathan was the one in the suit vowing unconditional commitment together from this day forward. However, I can already see that marriage only succeeds when you have support from all the people who have loved you into being the person you are. Nathan has been loving me and shaping me for a few years, but my aunts, uncles, parents, and brothers have already spent a lifetime shaping me into the person who is able to stand at the altar and confidently say that I am ready and willing "til death do us part." So now, I can see God's hand working through them. They truly were the glue that held this day together!

So, yes, we are big wedding people. I thought if I was lucky, I would see the silver lining of this pandemic wedding by the time June 13, 2021 rolls around, and instead it only took me until June 14, 2020. I got to talk to every one of our guests. I got to actually eat the wood-fired pizza at my own wedding. I got to sit in the backyard of my godparents' house, in my Wisconsin hometown, with four of my closest friends from college, in a wedding dress. I got to have fifty of our most important people in the church that I grew up in. I got to marry my absolute favorite person. I'm not just looking for silver linings anymore. The whole day was just perfectly golden.

The Tuskegee Study: Overcoming Racial Disparities in Vaccinations and Rebuilding the Trust of Black Americans

Balaraman Kalyanaraman, PhD

Dr. Kalanaraman, who was a graduate student in Alabama soon after the world became aware of the horrific studies at Tuskegee, wrote about how the racial injustice of the clinical trial has a lingering and dangerous effect.

"Injustice anywhere is a threat to justice everywhere. We are caught in an inescapable network of mutuality, tied in a single garment of destiny. Whatever affects one directly, affects all indirectly."
—Dr. Martin Luther King, Jr.

Racial disparity in vaccination is a sensitive topic. I am not an expert in this area; however, I want to address this issue because it is timely and a matter of life and death with COVID-19.

Black Americans are at increased risk of contracting SARS-CoV-2, nearly five times more likely to be hospitalized from COVID-19, and twice as likely to die from it as compared with white Americans. In the past, safe and effective vaccines saved millions of lives against pandemic viruses, yet the perception on vaccines and vaccinations remains varied among different groups struggling to decide whether to get vaccinated. Many people have lingering doubts about vaccine safety and even the motives behind vaccination. People have either forgotten about the Tuskegee Study or never heard of it. Reopening old wounds is not my objective, but I believe that knowing about and contemplating events of injustice in history make all of us better and will ensure that such acts are never repeated. Accurate information empowers people to make informed decisions. Encouraging Black American participation in vaccination, especially during the COVID-19 pandemic, should be a top priority.

Tuskegee Syphilis Study (1932-1972)

Tuskegee is in Macon County, Alabama, about 120 miles southeast of Birmingham. I was a graduate student in chemistry from 1974 to 1978 at the University of Alabama in Tuscaloosa, which is about 140 miles west of Tuskegee. The news about the Tuskegee Study broke in 1972. Having newly arrived from India in the midst of it all, I was clueless; I did not even know where Tuskegee was, let alone anything about the Tuskegee Study.

I found out about Tuskegee after I became a fan of

Lionel Richie (of The Commodores). Richie was born in Tuskegee, completing his undergraduate degree in economics at the Tuskegee Institute. The song "Easy (Like Sunday Morning)" is still one of my favorites, especially on Sundays. The real implications of the Tuskegee Study dawned on me only a few weeks ago, when I was watching a Sunday morning program discussing COVID-19 vaccinations, and why Black Americans are skeptical, suspicious, and even fearful of vaccines. The reason for their mistrust in vaccines? *Well, Tuskegee always looms large in their minds.*

What exactly was the Tuskegee Study? Nearly ninety years ago, the US Public Health Service began a clinical study in Tuskegee in which they enrolled six hundred Black men with and without syphilis. Many were enticed to participate with incentives such as free medical exams and meals, and even burial insurance. There was no informed consent. These men were not aware that they were participating in a study about syphilis; rather, they were told they would be treated for "bad blood," the local term for various ailments ranging from fatigue and anemia to syphilis. When the study began in 1932, there was no known treatment for syphilis. Thirteen years later, penicillin became the standard treatment for syphilis, yet it was withheld from the subjects who were infected. When asked why the study was not halted after determining that penicillin cured syphilis, the answer was: *Never again would they find such a cohort of "untreated" syphilis patients for medical information on organ damage.*

As a result, many untreated men died of syphilis, and

others suffered severe syphilis-related cardiovascular and neurological complications that persisted for years.

The legacy of the exploitive and unethical Tuskegee Study contributed to racial disparities in healthcare utilization and has had a long-lasting negative impact on the willingness of Black Americans to participate in clinical trials or vaccinations.

Increasing the participation of Black Americans in clinical trials and vaccinations

How can healthcare professionals dispel suspicions about clinical trials and vaccines, and regain the trust of Black Americans in vaccination? Finding a way for Black Americans to get past medical mistrust involves accurate and credible messaging as to why participation is important.

Diseases have disparate impacts on people depending on gender, race, ethnicity, age, and related factors, and drugs often exert different effects in different people. This is a whole new area of science known as pharmacogenetics—the science that reveals how genetic factors affect reactions to drugs and vaccinations. Thus, research protocols for clinical trials should include women, Black/African Americans, Hispanics/Latinx, and other racial and ethnic minorities in addition to white men. To ensure no group experiences untoward side effects in response to drug treatment, it is also necessary to increase the number of participants in each group.

Motivation to participate in clinical trials is often

personal and is triggered by different events in people's lives. This is where science can help. Sharing clinical success stories of scientific discoveries revolutionizing treatment of sickle cell disease, which predominantly affects people of African descent, is definitely encouraging! Most people know what DNA is and why it is important in life. That editing and correcting one error in the DNA of sickle cell patients could become a treatment or even a cure for this disease is likely to resonate better. This discovery was made possible because of participation in clinical trials.

As for vaccines, 1) communicate the best available, credible science on vaccine safety and the risks vs. benefits of vaccination; 2) explain how the vaccine was developed and managed with independent oversight and advisory groups; and 3) empower by providing available data from pharmaceutical companies on their trial protocols. Big pharmaceutical companies received our tax dollars to develop COVID-19 vaccines.

To lessen this disparity and empower people to make informed decisions, healthcare professionals must share accurate information from trusted sources.

Integrating the Humanities into Medical Education

Bruce H. Campbell, MD, FACS

Dr. Campbell created this essay for an issue about the humanities. He shares that building observational and representational skills through the humanities can offer a pathway into more empathetic and effective patient care.

"Stories are the primordial means through which we make sense of, and convey the meaning of, our lives."
—Rita Charon and Craig Irvine

My medical student group gathered to debrief and discuss their very first experiences observing physicians caring for patients. One student presented a case of a teenager she saw in her clinical mentor's office with mild muscle aches. This teen had a couple of relatives who were afflicted with a rare, devastating inherited disease. The boy's few vague symptoms could, possibly, represent the disorder's very earliest manifestations. Or the symptoms might be nothing at all.

"What did you decide to do?" I asked.

"We told him to exercise and take Advil. We also ordered genetic testing and asked him to come back in a few weeks to check the results."

"Thanks. That was a very complete presentation," I responded. "Does anyone have any questions?" Someone wanted to know more about the genetic testing. Someone else asked about other potential diagnoses. We discussed those.

"A couple more questions," I said. "Did the doctor find out how all this might be affecting the young man? Is he aware that he might have the same disease his relatives have? What do you think is going on inside his head?"

The student's eyes widened. "I don't know. We didn't ask."

I could not help but wonder whether the students might have been more curious about this teenager's underlying story had they heard this example a few months *before* they started medical school instead of a few months *after*.

Empathy levels will decrease. How soon does that happen?

In this profession, we lose our "vicarious empathy," or *our ability to have a visceral empathic response to another person's stressful experience*, very early on. A

2008 study from the University of Arkansas for Medical Sciences (UAMS) demonstrated significant drops in empathy during medical school, especially during the first and third years. Men (like me) who chose surgical specialties (also, like me) had the greatest loss of vicarious empathy.

Of course, no one plans to jettison their empathy along the way from being a normal person to becoming a physician. The losses likely occur as we seek to model ourselves after people who are a step or two ahead of us along the path. When I talk to first year students in MCW's Healer's Art course, they all affirm that they will listen to their patients, think first and foremost of the patient's well-being, and always act with justice and equanimity. Yet, some would not recognize the people that they will become once they emerge, transformed, from residency a few years later.

Professionalism vs. Humanism

How do we address this nearly imperceptible transformation from empathic layperson to crusty physician?

One way is to reflect on the values of both "Professionalism" and "Humanism." In medical schools, we strive to nurture professionals, which we might define as "physicians with attributes, skills, and demeanors with which they will practice high-quality medicine with integrity and empathy." This is, of course, an admirable goal. "Humanism," on the other hand, is broader than professionalism. These are the qualities we hope every physician brings to the table from childhood and that must be nurtured and enhanced, not lost, throughout the process of becoming a physician.

This is where integrating the humanities into medical education and training comes in.

Broadly defined, the medical humanities are interdisciplinary endeavors that draw on the creative and intellectual strengths of diverse disciplines, including the humanities, social science, and the arts in pursuit of becoming a good physician. They tap into literature, art, dance, creative writing, drama, dance, film, music, philosophy, ethical decision-making, anthropology, and history. It's basically the intersection of *Medicine* with *Everything Creative*. The goal is to draw on the humanities to expand a physician's capacity to be humanistic, compassionate, and empathetic.

Think of an example from your own life:

Remember a novel you read and loved in high school. If the narrative grabbed you, you dove into the protagonist's story and couldn't put the book down. You didn't worry that you "cared too much" for the protagonist or their struggles. You actively attempted to understand what each character was thinking, and you figured out why they did the things they did, even when their actions might have seemed, at first, inexplicable. Your heart rate soared when you anticipated danger, and you wiped your eyes when they suffered. Your blood boiled when they were betrayed. When you finished the book, you encapsulated the arc of the story and shared it with your best friend. You paid attention to the story. You were able to retell it to others. It changed you.

Ideally, as physicians, we should be similarly curious and fearless as we delve into our patient's narratives. We safely encountered narratives in the library. We should be able to do it at the bedside, as well. Right?

Yeah, but does reading a novel really make me a better doctor?

It does, actually. In a 2013 article in *Science* entitled, "Reading Literary Fiction Improves Theory of the Mind," the authors studied people who read literary fiction, popular fiction, nonfiction, or nothing at all. They discovered that those who read literary fiction demonstrated improved "theory of the mind," that is, *"the human capacity to comprehend that other people hold beliefs and desires and that these may differ from one's own beliefs and desires."* The article further showed that the same readers had stronger "theory of the mind" in both *cognitive* (the ability to understand others' beliefs and ideas) and *affective* (the ability to understand others' emotions or have empathy) realms. These were exactly the attributes that were lost during medical training in the UAMS study.

Narrative Medicine: Attention. Representation. Affiliation.

Rita Charon, MD, PhD, and her colleagues at Columbia University developed the field of Narrative Medicine over twenty years ago, bringing their "close reading" approach to clinics, classrooms, patients, ICUs, and bedsides. Participants first read and discuss a short story, poem, piece of artwork, or other creative work. Then for a few minutes, they each respond in writing to a simple but ambiguous prompt "in the shadow" of the piece they shared. Then they each read aloud what they have created and discuss as a group what they have learned through this process.

Dr. Charon teaches that these short, group-based exercises sharpen learners' listening capacities and drive the "self" to engage in new ways with the "other." "Reading and listening are muscular acts," Dr. Charon writes. "It makes us wonder about the spaces between the lines and forces us to join with the storyteller to enter the world they describe."

I have shared close reading exercises with MCW medical students, residents, and faculty over the years. These opportunities to read and write together have been gratifyingly well received. Other faculty, staff, and students have developed programs featuring writing, storytelling, art, improv, music, and other creative endeavors.

Many students embrace these approaches, and faculty members deeply enjoy the engagement, but we still struggle, as have many other medical schools, to truly integrate the humanities into medical education for all our trainees.

Where do we begin to integrate the humanities into medical education?

In 2020, the Association of American Medical Colleges (AAMC) released a report on the Fundamental Role of Arts and Humanities in Medical Education. The AAMC recognizes that the "arts and humanities are essential to the human experience," and by "integrating arts and humanities throughout medical education, trainees and physicians can learn to be better observers and interpreters." The report offers resources and examples for students and educators who want to explore the topic. As Deepthiman Gowda, MD, the Assistant Dean for Medical Education at the Kaiser Permanente Bernard J. Tyson School of Medicine has said, "Humanities have a role in addressing the problems in healthcare."

There is, too often, a chasm between physicians and patients, and medical training, paradoxically, seems to widen that chasm. The humanities, well used, can assist in bridging this gap. Substantively integrating the humanities into medical education could sustain and enhance the empathy students bring to medical training and provide them with tools to remain resilient, deeply compassionate, and attentive caregivers.

Curricular change is hard. We will know we have succeeded when our youngest colleagues hold onto their empathy even when it sometimes seems easier to let it go.

Hugs in Grand Rapids

Wendy Peltier, MD

*As the travel restrictions were being slowly lifted,
Dr. Peltier took a trip home to see her family.
Hugs were important.*

The trip to Grand Rapids is five hours when there is
no Chicago traffic. For me, the time is usually filled with
road trip snacks, juggling kids' requests from the back
seat, and trying to steal a few moments in a magazine
without getting carsick while my husband drives. This
February, it was much different.

I tried to keep myself from getting excited the week
before, knowing that at any moment, there might be cause
to cancel. I had already received my two vaccine doses, so
I was less worried about my COVID-19 test results, but I
wanted to be doubly sure to travel safely. I found myself
more worried about a kid requiring quarantine, a caregiver

falling sick, or a dreaded Wisconsin snowstorm forcing us to reschedule.

When the day finally arrived, I was giddy. On the road, I smiled between the tears as my car crossed into Illinois. I marveled at how this once familiar road now seemed foreign and crisply real. It was just me, my "Faves" playlist on Spotify, a hot mug of coffee, and an unnerving sense of being too close to big semi-trucks. *Could it really be over a year since I had seen my folks? Could it really be that I would have four uninterrupted days to share with them, just the three of us?*

It seemed I processed the year of the pandemic as the miles ticked away.

This time of solitude in the car brought waves of relief, joy, gratitude . . . but also guilt. I felt keenly aware that so many in my community, our nation, and the world, no longer had this opportunity. For those of you with aging parents, it's all too familiar that the gnawing fear of a serious health issue might arise in normal times. This year of COVID-19 amplified that considerably for us and led my family to forgo highly anticipated time together, such as our "do-not-miss" Fourth of July gala at the summer cabin, holiday gatherings, and my mom's eightieth birthday celebration. Like so many of my colleagues in healthcare and education, we just couldn't take the risk of being together.

Although we connected regularly by telephone and Zoom calls, it felt insufficient for the magnitude of what we were facing with the pandemic. We tried to be positive on those calls, but much of the worry and fear we were experiencing was left unspoken. We tried to lift each other up and connect, but there was always a distance created by the ever-present technology snafus, "noises" in the household, and pressing deadlines to meet. Throughout the year, the stilted interactions became normalized, and it became harder to remember the last moments we were actually together.

This trip was so different for me, compared to the many other times having been on this same road. I brought with me the immense sense of relief that my parents had also been vaccinated. We were safe to be together. As Michigan got closer, I realized how many nights I had lain awake worrying about what might happen should one of my parents contract the virus. In caring for families at the hospital with a loved one ill or dying from COVID-19 in isolation, it felt so close . . . *This could be us, my family.*

I finally arrived. That first big bear hug was pretty incredible. It was hard to let go. I had that same heightened sense of reality, of all my senses being activated at once by the familiar smell of home, the beauty of the space, and the overwhelming sense of relief. I think my folks felt that, too.

Then, the relaxation and fun began. I was so touched by how my mom made all my favorite foods without asking, how much I enjoyed being part of activities that had filled their daily lives during this long quarantine, and how quickly we settled into our old habits of being together. The weekend was filled with reconnecting and taking time to just relax in each other's company. The gnawing feeling in my stomach began to lessen, and I felt a renewed sense of strength and energy. I felt lucky.

On the ride back to Wisconsin, I felt lighter, and a bit more normal again.

It was obviously hard to leave, but I left with the knowledge we would be together again soon. It seemed I could finally believe that the worst of the pandemic was over. It was time to look ahead to new challenges and opportunities, both at work and for my Wisconsin family. It was time to focus on healing rather than simply surviving.

As I write about this experience, I sincerely hope that similar reunions will be coming for so many of my friends, colleagues, and extended family as we look to recover from the COVID-19 pandemic. I hope we also continue to seek opportunities to honor and support families who have lost loved ones during this tumultuous time. And that when it's truly safe to do so, hugs will abound!

Sixteen Months

Doris Larson

Ms. Larson, the mother of Wendy Peltier, MD, wrote this poem in response to the family trip to visit her.

How do you measure
A sixteen-month absence
From a beloved daughter?

In Pride
For a caring physician
Dedicated to her patients.

In Fear
For her safety
Daily in the hospital.

In Gratitude
For her supportive husband
And loving sons.

In Anxiety
For the spread of COVID
Surrounding us all.

In Hope
For a vaccinated world
Forever changed.

In Joy
For the daughter's visit.
The restorative power of hugs.

Community Reflections: If you could travel back to January 1, 2020, what would you want to tell your former self?

Cathy Brummer in Pediatrics submitted this response:
Plans change . . . be flexible.

Kathryn Golab from Wisconsin Diagnostic Laboratories submitted this response:
This year will be completely different than anything you have ever experienced, and it will change you for the better. Don't panic, take a deep breath, and keep putting one foot in front of the other.

Community Reflections: What do you hope we all learn from this experience?

An anonymous medical student submitted this response:
In our life after this pandemic, I really hope the feeling of community sticks. I have been greeted on my runs and walks more in the last two months than probably ever before. There is an understanding that we are all going through the same thing, and people are going out of their way to check in with neighbors and friends. I hope that continues into the future. As Americans, we are

individualistic and self-centered. I hope that experiencing a time where we are forced to think about the benefit of the community before ourselves will teach us how important it is to serve and care for our communities.

Kathlyn Fletcher, MD, submitted this response:

I hope that we learn the value of being together. I find myself looking back longingly on rather ordinary gatherings that I used to host fairly often. I miss laughing with friends and extended family—the value of being with people we choose. I also hope to remember the moments of joy that would not have happened in my pre-COVID-19 life. Watching an episode of West Wing each night with my teenage daughter. Sitting next to my ten-year-old son as he works. Preparing and eating actual family dinner—the value of being with family. I love the way our community has shown that we are all in this together. Signs, texts, drive-by parades, food, prayers and good wishes—being together in spirit.

Embrace. It is Time.

Mary Sellars

Ms. Sellars, daughter of MCW faculty member Sandra Pfister, PhD, wrote this poem after Sandra's mother passed away in 2008.

The quiet blooming of a tulip
The flowing death of sunshine rays
It is time

The melancholy calls of the tall golden gates
and celestial key
It is time

I am not the person to hold on
It is autumn's falling leaves

Embrace your reflection in the mirror
Roaring past all your tales

Embrace
It is time

For this to end
Let it come like winter blooms

It is time

Embrace

It is time

Contributors

Himanshu Agrawal, MD, DF-APA, is an Assistant Professor in the Department of Psychiatry and Behavioral Health at MCW and co-director of the psychiatry clerkship. He serves as a small group facilitator in the Kern REACH curriculum.

Paul A. Bergl, MD, was an Assistant Professor of Medicine in Pulmonary, Critical Care, and Sleep Medicine at MCW. He is now a critical care physician with Gundersen Health in La Crosse, WI.

Bruce H. Campbell, MD, FACS, is a Professor of Otolaryngology & Communication Sciences and is on the faculty of the Center for Bioethics & Medical Humanities at MCW. He is on the Faculty Pillar of the Robert D. and Patricia E. Kern Institute for the Transformation of Medical Education. He serves as the Editor-in-Chief of the *Transformational Times*.

David A. Campbell, MD, graduated from the MCW otolaryngology residency in 2021. He is currently the Head and Neck Oncology - Microvascular Reconstructive

Surgery fellow at the Icahn School of Medicine at Mt. Sinai in New York City.

Mario Castellanos, MD, graduated from MCW-Milwaukee in 2021. He is currently a resident in the Harvard Affiliated Emergency Medicine Residency at Mass General Brigham.

Olivia Davies, MD, graduated from MCW-Milwaukee in 2021. She is currently a resident in the Harvard Combined Dermatology Residency Program. As a medical student, she was an Associate Editor of the *Transformational Times*.

Christopher Davis, MD, MPH, is an Assistant Professor of Surgery (Trauma and Acute Care Surgery) at MCW. He is a faculty member of the Community and Institutional Engagement Pillar of the Robert D. and Patricia E. Kern Institute for the Transformation of Medical Education.

Catherine (Cassie) Ferguson, MD, is an Associate Professor of Pediatrics (Emergency Medicine) at MCW. She is the Associate Director of the Robert D. and Patricia E. Kern Institute for the Transformation of Medical Education and the founding director of the Student Pillar. She leads the MCW M1 and M2 REACH curriculum focused on promoting wellness.

José Franco, MD, is a Professor of Medicine and Pediatrics in the Division of Gastroenterology and Hepatology, founding Director of the Cross Pillar, of the Robert D. and Patricia E. Kern Institute for the

Transformation of Medical Education and now Interim Senior Associate Dean for Academic Affairs at MCW.

Camille B. Garrison, MD, is Assistant Professor of Family and Community Medicine. Dr. Garrison works and teaches in the Columbia-St. Mary's Family Health Center.

Ashley M. Hines was the Diversity and Inclusion Manager in the MCW Office of Diversity and Inclusion. She is now the Director of Diversity and Inclusion at Advocate Aurora Health.

Ana Istrate, MD, MS, is a resident in the Internal Medicine Residency Program at MCW.

Sherréa Jones, PhD, a medical student at MCW-Milwaukee.

Adina Kalet, MD, MPH, is Director of the Robert D. and Patricia E. Kern Institute for the Transformation of Medical Education and holder of the Stephen and Shelagh Roell Endowed Chair at the Medical College of Wisconsin. She is an editor of the *Transformational Times*.

Balaraman Kalyanaraman, PhD, is Professor and Chair of the Department of Biophysics at MCW.

Joseph E. Kerschner, MD, FACS, FAAP, is the Provost, Executive Vice President, and Dean of the School of Medicine at MCW.

Sophia Kiernan is a medical student at MCW-Milwaukee. She is part of the Kern Institute's Student Physician Networking Program.

Doris Larson, who contributed a poem, is the mother of Wendy Peltier, MD.

Chase LaRue is a medical student at MCW-Milwaukee. He is part of the MedMoth Planning Team.

Karen Marcdante, MD, is a Professor of Pediatrics (Critical Care) at MCW. She is Director of the Human Centered Design Lab and serves on the Kinetic3 Teaching Academy Steering Committee and on the Faculty Pillar of the Robert D. and Patricia E. Kern Institute for the Transformation of Medical Education.

Michelle Minikel, MD, is a Family Physician and practices through Bellin Health in Green Bay, WI. She leads the Clínica Hispana.

Keng Moua is a medical student at MCW-Milwaukee.

David Nelson, PhD, MS, is an Associate Professor of Family and Community Medicine at MCW. He serves on the board of Friedens Community Ministries, a local network of food pantries working to end hunger in the community.

Loren Nunley, MD, MBA, is an Infectious Diseases specialist working in the Chicago metropolitan area. He graduated from the MCW Infectious Diseases fellowship in 2021.

Wendy Peltier, MD, is an Associate Professor of Medicine and Neurology in the Division of Geriatric and Palliative Medicine at MCW. She is on the Faculty Pillar of the Robert D. and Patricia E. Kern Institute for the Transformation of Medical Education. She serves as an editor of the *Transformational Times.*

Sandra Pfister, PhD, is a Professor of Pharmacology and Toxicology at MCW. She is Interim Director of the Clinical Learning Environment Pillar and serves on the Faculty Pillar of the Robert D. and Patricia E. Kern Institute for the Transformation of Medical Education.

Anglea Polcyn, MS, is a thanatologist who works as a bereavement coordinator at Froedtert & MCW.

Katherine A. (Katie) Recka, MD, is an Associate Professor of Medicine in the Division of Geriatric and Palliative Medicine at MCW. She currently serves as the Section Chief for the Palliative Service at the Zablocki VAMC.

Victor Redmon, MD, is a resident in the MCW combined medicine and pediatrics residency program. He is currently a chief resident.

Maya Saravanan is a medical student at MCW-Milwaukee.

Megan L. Schultz, MD, MA, is an Assistant Professor of Pediatrics (Emergency Medicine) at MCW.

Mark D. Schwartz, MD, is a Professor of Medicine and Population Health, Vice Chair for Education and Faculty Affairs, Department of Population Health, New York University Grossman School of Medicine. He leads pre- and post-doctoral fellowship programs in population health and health policy.

Mary Sellars, who contributed a poem, is the daughter of Sandra Pfister, PhD.

Leroy J. Seymour, MD, MS, is a resident in the Internal Medicine Residency Program at MCW.

Malika Siker, MD, is an Associate Professor of Radiation Oncology and the Associate Dean for Student Inclusion and Diversity at MCW.

Christopher Stawski, PhD, is Senior Program Director and Senior Fellow of the Kern Family Foundation, a member of the Student Pillar and the Philosophies of Medical Education Transformation Lab (P-MeTL) of the Robert D. and Patricia E. Kern Institute for the Transformation of Medical Education, and a member of multiple workgroups of the Kern National Network for Caring and Character in Medicine.

Hayden Swartz is a medical student at MCW-Central Wisconsin.

Jake Taxis, MDiv, BCC, is a Lutheran Minister and dedicated chaplain for the Palliative Care Team at Froedtert Hospital.

Permissions

Each essay in this volume was published in the *Transformational Times* newsletter and the authors have provided permission to have their work reprinted here. Individuals identified by name have provided permission to the essayist to do so.

In addition, the following essays were also published previously in other formats:

Garrison, Camille B, "The Lonely Only: Physician Reflections on Race, Bias, and Residency Program Leadership." *Family Medicine* 2019 Jan;51(1):59-60. doi: 10.22454/FamMed.2019.339526. Copyright Society of Teachers of Family Medicine. Used by permission.

"Microaggression." Reproduced with permission from Campbell, Bruce H. *A Fullness of Uncertain Significance: Stories of Surgery, Clarity, & Grace.* Waukesha WI, Ten16 Press, 2021.

Acknowledgements

This book would not have been possible without the support and hard work of many people:

Thank you to the Kern Family Foundation for its vision and support, both of the Kern Institute and this project.

Thank you to the *Transformational Times* essayists, poets, and visual artists who fearlessly created and submitted their insightful pieces during these difficult months. We are more awestruck each time we revisit your work.

Thank you to the people in the administration of the Medical College of Wisconsin who believed in what we were trying to do and trusted us to do it.

Thank you to the talented team at Orange Hat Publishing | Ten16 Press who helped take this book from idea to reality in an incredibly short time, especially publisher Shannon Ishizaki, art director Kaeley Dunteman, and editor Jenna Zerbel.

The *Transformational Times* Editorial Team:
Bruce H. Campbell, MD, FACS
Kathlyn Fletcher, MD, MA
Adina Kalet, MD, MPH
Wendy Peltier, MD

Associate Editors (2020-2021):
Olivia Davies
Scott Lamm
Eileen Peterson
Sarah Torres
Anna Visser

Production Editors:
Julia Schmitt
Erin Weileder

Selections Editor:
Rachel Keane